Dreams, Symbols & Homeopathy

Dreams, Symbols & Homeopathy

Archetypal Dimensions of Healing

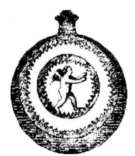

Jane Cicchetti

North Atlantic Books
Berkeley, California

Homeopathic Educational Services
Berkeley, California

This book is dedicated to my mother.

Published by
North Atlantic Books
P.O. Box 12327
Berkeley, California 94712

and
Homeopathic Educational Services
2124 Kittredge Street #2
Berkeley, California 94704

Cover and text design by Susan Quasha
Printed in Canada

Dreams, Symbols and Homeopathy: Archetypal Dimensions of Healing is sponsored by the Society for the Study of Native Arts and Sciences, a nonprofit educational corporation whose goals are to develop an educational and cross-cultural perspective linking various scientific, social, and artistic fields; to nurture a holistic view of arts, sciences, humanities, and healing; and to publish and distribute literature on the relationship of mind, body, and nature.

North Atlantic Books' publications are available through most bookstores. For further information, visit our Web site at www.northatlanticbooks.com or call 800-733-3000.

ISBN-13: 978-1-55643-436-5

Library of Congress Cataloging-in-Publication Data

Cicchetti, Jane, 1943-
   Dreams, symbols, and homeopathy : archetypal dimensions of healing /
by Jane Cicchetti.
        p. ; cm.
Includes bibliographical references and index.
   ISBN 1-55643-436-7
   1. Homeopathy—Philosophy. 2. Dreams. 3. Healing—Psychological
aspects. 4. Symbolism (Psychology) 5. Archetype (Psychology) 6.
Jungian psychology. 7. Medicine and psychology. 8. Mind and body.
   [DNLM: 1. Dreams. 2. Homeopathy—methods. 3. Jungian Theory. 4.
Mental Healing. WB 930 C568d 2003] I. Title.
   RX72.C53 2003
   615.5'32'01—dc21

2003006785

3 4 5 6 7 8 TRANS 13 12 11 10

Contents

About the Cover

The illustration on the cover is from a sixteenth-century woodcut and represents the legend of Charlemagne and the carline thistle. According to the legend, Charlemagne's army was suffering from a terrible plague that killed many of his men. Charlemagne prayed for help, and an angel appeared to him in his sleep. Shooting a bolt from a crossbow, the angel told Charlemagne that where the bolt landed would mark a plant that he could use to cure his men. When Charlemagne awoke, he found a plant with a crossbow bolt through its root. With this root, he was able to cure his soldiers of the plague.

The carline thistle *(Carlina vulgaris)* is mentioned by the ancient herbalist Culpepper as capable of curing the plague.

Preface

The purpose of this book is to help homeopaths and others interested in the relationship between the psyche and healing to use dreams and symbols in their work. Because Carl Jung was instrumental in developing a systematic approach to dreams, his view of the psyche plays an important role. It is my hope that the information contained herein will enhance the understanding of the mind-body relationship and be of assistance in situations where the cause of disease is deeply hidden or difficult to understand.

In order to stay as close to the source as possible, I have relied primarily on Jung's original works and secondarily on works written by two Jungian analysts who were very close to Jung: Edward Edinger and Marie-Louise von Franz.

None of this careful assimilation of Jung's work would have been possible without the guidance of Jungian analyst Walter Odajnyk, who read through much of the text and corrected any misconceptions I may have had about Jung's ideas. I am very grateful for his help.

Christopher Phillips, C.C.H., has generously shared with me his knowledge of the art of communication, so these sometimes difficult ideas could be more easily understood.

Many thanks are due to my homeopathic colleagues, Jan Scholten, T. Namaya, and Jean Pierre Jansen, for taking time from their busy lives to preview this work and adding constructive comments as it evolved. I would especially like to thank my dear friend and colleague Alize Timmerman, who has shared her knowledge of healing and homeopathy with me over the years and spent much time reviewing this material.

Dana Ullman enthusiastically took on this project for North Atlantic Books from its onset and has been a source of encouragement and inspiration along the way.

I would also like to thank Lisa Nolan, who cheerfully assisted me in every detail of working on this manuscript.

This book would not have been possible without the many people who have given permission to have their personal stories included. Although they must necessarily remain anonymous, I thank them all.

Jane Cicchetti

Introduction

I first met Jane Cicchetti many years ago at a seminar and immediately felt that she had a lot to contribute to the world of homeopathy and healing. At that time homeopathy was not ready to receive many of her ideas, as very few people in the field were working with information from the symbolic world. Even so, I felt very strongly that it was important for her to continue in the direction she was going and knew that if she developed her work with dreams and symbols, she would make an important and reliable contribution to the field.

Jane developed her ideas of how dreams, symbols, and Jung's concept of the psyche fit into homeopathy to a high degree and the result is this book.

Now, the time is right to open our eyes to a bigger picture of what is meant by healing, and her work will help us to do this.

One of the most interesting things about this book is that, along with practical information, it opens the reader's awareness of the archetypal levels of reality, thereby creating the opportunity for change. Not only does Jane give a massive amount of information about symbolism and its clinical application, but she also touches the reader's unconscious symbolic world.

From the very beginning, on reading the first chapter, I felt inspired. This book not only enriched my conscious awareness of the healing process but also enlivened my unconscious world. My dream world started to awaken, and I began to understand more about my dreams. The meaning of even very old dreams that I had previously not understood became clear.

From my point of view, this is what is most important about this book—that it leads one to understand the symbolic world from a personal perspective, thus enlivening the symbolic world and allowing it to be used in healing both oneself and others.

In homeopathy, we like to prescribe on the biggest totality that we can perceive. This book explains how we can perceive a larger picture of reality through the insight that dreams and symbols give us into the world of the unconscious.

This is the first book on homeopathy to give an in-depth understanding of the psyche and the world of dreams. Jane explains in minute detail how to use dreams in a way that allows homeopaths to prescribe remedies with a greater level of confidence and accuracy.

The first chapter gives us a historical view of the development of underlying beliefs about healing and distinguishes between two different philosophies of medicine, empiricism and rationalism. This helps the reader understand the underlying philosophy of homeopathy as compared to conventional medicine.

The second half of the book is an exploration of symbols in regards to remedies within the homeopathic materia medica. Here, Jane helps us to understand the relationship between substances and human consciousness. Mythological and archetypal symbolism are compared with provings and clinically known uses of remedies to help expand the homeopath's understanding of their curative effects. Her exploration of the symbolic meaning of the actual substance clarifies the information in the original provings.

The information in the chapter on the seven metals and the chapter on trees is a treat in itself, and will be of interest to those to whom homeopathy is unknown and to the professional homeopath.

The beautiful chapter on the role of the "internal saboteur" in healing helps to shed light on the problem of the patient who never moves forward in the healing process. This chapter is especially important because it gives the professional homeopath a deeper understanding of why certain patients are not helped by the indicated remedy.

I hope that this book touches you as deeply as it did me and that you also feel that you can grow from it and use it in your daily practice.

Alize Timmerman
THE HANN INSTITUTE
THE HAGUE, NETHERLANDS

PART I

Emergence of the Opposites

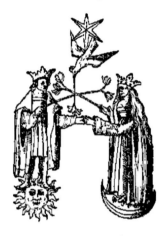

The Rosarium Philosophorum, *first printed in the second volume of* De Alchimia opuscula complura veterum philosophorum, Frankfurt 1550.

This alchemical woodcut can be seen as an illustration of opposites agreeing to be reconciled. Psychologist Carl Jung has said that as society becomes more and more chaotic, our only hope is for individuals to make a conscious consolidation of opposite forces within themselves to serve as a counterbalance. Medicine can play an important role in helping individuals to make this transformation, if it recognizes the existence of its own inner conflicts and finds a way to resolve them.

This first section will cover the need for integration of the schism between empiricism and rationalism and the opposition between symbolic wisdom and scientific rationalism in medicine. It will also introduce homeopathy as a method of treatment that addresses the whole person and has the potential to use information from both the symbolic and rational realms. Finally, this section will explore the problem of scientific rationalism when addressing the mind-body relationship and propose a method for reconciling opposing philosophies in medicine.

CHAPTER ONE

Archetypal Dimensions of Healing
A New Paradigm for Medicine

Medicinal herbs, ceremonies, and myths of healing have been an important part of the human experience since we first walked the earth. The quest for healing lies so deeply within the human psyche that it may even predate our own species. It is now known that many primates use healing plants as a part of their diet. Chimpanzees and gorillas seek out and use medicinal plants, and a skeleton of a Neanderthal has been found buried with medicinal plants encircling his body.

The impulse toward healing and wholeness is a fundamental instinct of life that cannot be satisfied solely through one medical system or another, as it belongs to the inner life of the individual and is part of the collective human experience. To confine this realm to the profession of medicine, and especially one standard of institutionalized medical care, is to dissect and severely limit an essential aspect of life.

The institutionalization of medicine is, however, not the cause, but a symptom of the dilemma in which we presently find ourselves. It is symptomatic of the fragmentation that human beings are experiencing due to the reductionist tendency of logic and a commitment to rational thinking that has developed over the ages. In *Wholeness and the Implicate Order,* written in 1980, physicist David Bohm refers to the problems caused by the illusion that life exists in fragments:

> *The notion that all these fragments are separately existent is evidently an illusion, and this illusion cannot do other than lead to endless conflict and confusion. Indeed, the attempt to live according to the notion that the fragments are really separate is, in essence, what has led to the growing series of extremely urgent crises that is confronting us today.*

*Thus, as is now well known, this way of life has brought about pollu-
tion, destruction of the balance of nature, over-population, world-wide
economic and political disorder, and the creation of an overall environment that is neither physically nor mentally healthy for most of the
people who have to live in it. Individually there has developed a wide-
spread feeling of helplessness and despair, in the face of what seems to be
an overwhelming mass of disparate social forces, going beyond the control
and even the comprehension of the human beings who are caught up in it.*[1]

The challenge of this time is to integrate a sense of wholeness into the
divisionary, rational approach to life. This entails retrieving feminine power
that has been dominated by a patriarchal attitude, bringing spirit back into
an era overwhelmed by materialism, and allowing the mystical to take a
place within the rational.

A time where there is need of such great transformation requires the
ability to grow and adapt to rapidly changing conditions. This increases the
amount of stress, which manifests in different types of health problems.

Along with the stressful nature of the times, other factors have affected
our health and well-being. Technological advances, created without considering their effect on the greater whole, have caused problems of alienation
and toxicity. Methods of farming and mining, implemented without concern for the environment, have resulted in ecological disasters that threaten
millions of people who live in nearby areas and, in some cases, are creating
new and dangerous breeds of bacteria. Human beings have become petri
dishes for these new strains of viruses and bacteria, and our overcrowded
global community is in danger of devastating epidemics from more and
more horrific diseases. At the end of her encyclopedic book on the development of new infectious diseases, *The Coming Plague*, health and science
writer Laurie Garrett leaves us with this chilling warning:

*While the human race battles itself, fighting over ever more crowded
turf and scarcer resources, the advantage moves to the microbes' court.
They are our predators and they will be victorious if we,* Homo sapiens
*do not learn how to live in a rational global village that affords the
microbes few opportunities.*

It's either that or we brace ourselves for the coming plague.[2]

From a medical perspective, these are problems that can no longer be
solved by the present standard of medicine. They have been caused by
fragmentation and must be addressed by systems of medicine that integrate

a vision of wholeness into technological advances. This is not to say that we should discard these advances. What is required is a new paradigm that allows the mystery of healing and the awareness of wholeness to enter into the practice of modern medicine. One vehicle to help us move toward this integration is the use of dreams.

Dreams are the doorway to the symbolic realm of the psyche—a powerful force underlying human consciousness. It is an ancient and primeval realm, containing the history of life on this planet and perhaps even beyond. To walk through this door can be frightening, for this realm contains fears and superstitions that mankind has long desired to control as we moved out of the primal oneness with nature, but it can also be rewarding.

The memory of the primal oneness is in each of us, as we have all experienced it in infancy. As we develop into adulthood we gain a sense of self or ego that differentiates us from the rest of our experience. It is a necessary separation—those who do not achieve it are unable to function optimally in life.

After achieving a differentiated sense of self, there is another equally important phase that must follow, and that is the return to the source that once nourished us. It is a phase of development that allows for perception of a greater reality than the ego while still maintaining a sense of separation. Unfortunately, few people make the journey into this second phase of development.

We are at a juncture in time, however, in which it is necessary for human beings at large to move into this phase of development. This development requires integration of a sense of wholeness into the differentiated, rational approach to life. This is not a return to the primitive, but a synthesis between the symbolic and the rational realms that allows for an entirely new way of thinking. It is to this end that a new paradigm of medicine is needed, for the health of human beings and the planet depends upon this integration.

Dreams are the vehicle through which this second phase of development can be made, as they allow for a return to the source while still maintaining a sense of self. They help us to reconnect with the body, our instinctual self, and the wisdom accumulated within human consciousness from the time of our first ancestors. Dreams are an essential component in healing, an attempt on the part of the organism to heal itself directly or through indications of what is needed in order to heal. The use of dreams in medicine is not a retreat into fantasy; it is a necessary adjustment to a trend that has gone too far.

Fortunately, our ability to connect with the depths of our inner selves is not lost, but simply slumbering, unattended. Through dreams, myths, and symbols, human beings still have the capacity to reach into the inner realm of consciousness and retrieve what has been lost in man's search for his rational self.

In order to create a background for the use of dreams in healing in general, and more specifically in homeopathy, this chapter will cover the development of human consciousness as it moved from the primeval state of oneness with nature to its more detached, rational stage. It will then go into a necessarily brief recap of two historically antagonistic philosophical views in medicine—empiricism and rationalism. After this, we will make a huge, feet-first leap—directly into an experience of the archetypal realm of dreams, an experience that will, ideally, imbue the reader with the desire to further pursue this adventure.

Emerging from Oneness

Humanity was once immersed in the womb of Mother Earth through the world of dreams, symbols, and mythology. In order to mature, humanity needed to leave her womb and evolve the use of rational thought. Through rational thinking, humans were able to separate and analyze pieces of reality. This stage, though necessary, led to the present-day detachment of the mind from the emotions, spirit, and wholeness in general.

Our early ancestors understood the phenomena of the world around them as manifestations of gods and goddesses. Nature was beneficent and frightening at the same time. Thunderstorms, solar eclipses, and even the movement of celestial bodies were perceived as magical events that needed to be worshipped for their great power. Our ancestors were clearly aware that they were at the mercy of weather patterns and the presence or absence of food sources. Myths explained these events, and rituals were performed to assuage these powers. Men and women lived lives that were closely attuned to nature. They understood that they were not separate from but intimately tied to all of the natural events of the Earth. The physicians of the time were as often women as men and were respected as conduits for the gods and sources of knowledge of nature's healing gifts. For thousands of years, humankind lived in this relationship to nature.

For a period of about five hundred years, the mythological world met with the emergence of rational thought, resulting in the rich culture of ancient Greece. Lasting from approximately 490 B.C. to A.D. 27, the classical

Greek period was a time of inspired balance between logos and mythos. This period gave rise to highly creative developments in philosophy, art, and science, including medicine. This culture developed the roots of Western medicine, the Aesculapian medicine of Hippocrates. Aesculapian medicine was a combination of scientific medicine, hygiene, and the use of the imagination and spirit. The Aesclepion, the ancient medical school and hospital on the island of Kos, boasted sleep temples where patients would await the dreams of Aesculapius, the god of healing, while other areas of the hospital were reserved for surgery and herbal treatments. In a feat that is unique in the history of medicine, the Greek physicians were able to integrate the use of rationalism with empirical principles.

Several centuries after the golden age of Greece, this union of rational and intuitive knowledge was decimated by the rise of Christianity. What was once an exploration of the inner experience of humanity and the natural world was taken over by the authority of the church, which demanded faith and belief in the scriptures as the only road to the truth.

Around 1650, the worldview began to change again. It was a natural reaction against the oppression of the intellect by the church and also against the superstition that still dominated the human mind. In an attempt to overthrow these impediments, new philosophies and types of research began to emerge. Led by the discoveries of Isaac Newton that related natural occurrences to mathematics and the inquiries of philosophers such as René Descartes and John Locke, humanity began to take a more rational and scientific approach to religious, social, and political issues. These approaches in turn promoted a secular view of the world. The use of empirical evidence and the scientific method allowed for clear thinking, detached from the inner psychic world of emotion, and led to many of the great strides in technology and science, including developments in transportation, improved methods of farming, and technology such as the microscope, which helped extend the ability of the senses.

Medicine became increasingly institutionalized with the growing numbers of medical schools, hospitals, and regulations, while those who still worked with the remedies of nature were persecuted. A profession that once contained many women became dominated by the patriarchy, and a large number of these women, knowledgeable in midwifery and the use of healing plants, were burned as witches. The inner capacity for healing, present in nature and within the individual, was increasingly claimed by the professional physician and his patriarchal institutions.

Rationalist and Empiricist Medicine

As humans were moving toward a more rational and detached view of themselves and their environment, physicians were viewing health and disease from two disparate perspectives—empiricism and rationalism. The empiricist practitioners were more focused on observation of phenomena and the experience of practice, and rationalists were concerned with the development of structured knowledge through which they could view the mind and body. These two philosophies of medicine exist up to the present day, with rationalism dominating conventional medicine.

The empiricists' approach is holistic and accepts that healing comes from the inherent healing ability of the mind, body, and spirit. It is based on the hypothesis that a vital force, or *physis*, exists within a living organism, which generates both symptoms and healing. This belief is an important part of the philosophy known as vitalism. Systems that are primarily vitalist are homeopathy, chiropractic, acupuncture, and many Eastern healing modalities. Because empiricism attempts to perceive the patterns of knowledge within the structure of nature, it assumes that its conception of the structures will change with increasing information. Thus empiricism becomes a vehicle for scientifically exploring new ideas and finding creative solutions to problems in medicine and society.

Rationalists, who view the body from a purely materialistic perspective, vehemently reject the concept of physis. It should come as no surprise, therefore, that as human beings developed rational thought and rejected their deeper connection with spirit, rationalism dominated the medical arena, and empiricism, with its belief in vitalism, fell into disuse.

Seeing the body as a sophisticated machine, rational medicine considers the classification of knowledge of the body and disease to be of the utmost importance and the individual to be of secondary importance. Symptoms of most interest to the rationalist physician are those that are common to the disorder. Individual peculiarities are considered to be annoying anomalies that stand in the way of diagnosis. Research is done from autopsy, examination of tissue and fluid, and the study of chemistry and disease organisms. The resulting conclusions are then extrapolated onto diseases and the functioning of the body. Prognosis is usually determined by statistics.

Treatment in rational medicine, in addition to surgery, usually consists of a small number of general remedies, such as antibiotics, steroids, and other chemotherapeutic agents. These medicines are very widely used, and their efficacy diminishes over time, because disease organisms develop resistance to them. This leads to dependence on research by pharmaceutical companies, which are constantly looking for more powerful drugs.

Rationalism is responsible for many breakthroughs in the diagnosis of disease, development of advanced and life-saving surgical techniques, the discovery of new medications, and the invention of advanced medical technology. It has developed the capability to save lives that were once lost after traumatic accidents and to extend life through organ transplants and other sophisticated surgery. Without a doubt, rationalism has made a huge contribution to the advancement of medicine.

Rationalism has not, however, developed techniques that go to the core of the problem. It cannot cure chronic disease; rather, it treats symptoms of the disease, which often reappear as deeper and more insidious problems. Rationalist medicine fails to research the course of disease during treatment and lacks an understanding of the healing process. These failings are exacerbated by the fact that rationalist medicine has historically used its political clout to maintain a monopoly and has systematically denigrated principles of empiricist medicine, thus denying the public access to information and treatment that may be useful.

Proponents of empiricist medicine have historically been just as strongly against rationalism as the reverse. But, in the last century, empiricist medicine has not been as widely used as rationalism, despite the fact that, in many cases, empiricist physicians have gotten excellent results. Therefore empiricist medicine does not have the power to suppress other forms of treatment, as has the rationalist approach.

In his four-volume history of Western medicine, *Divided Legacy*, Harris Coulter writes of the reasons why empiricist medicine has not had as wide economic and political success as has rationalism:

> For the practice of medicine in a social setting involves much more than merely healing sick persons. The physician wants to do this, indeed, but he has other desiderata also. In particular, he wants to earn a respectable living from this activity and, in an undertaking so fraught with uncertainty, he may at times desire protection from the objects of his services.
>
> Medical doctrines, or "ideologies," as they may be called, appeal to physicians not only by their therapeutic potential but also by their ability to: (1) bind the medical profession together in a group which can resist social pressure, (2) create psychological distance between physician and the patient, and (3) enable the physician to make a satisfactory living.[3]

Coulter goes on to explain why rationalism serves these needs of the physician better than does empiricism, citing, among other characteristics, that the empiricists were often loners who were more interested in working with their patients and not very interested in forming professional organizations and political groups. This is characteristic of empiricist practitioners up to the present day, and although it is of great benefit to the individual patient, it does not create a profession that grows and thrives in a competitive market. Ultimately, empiricist medicine's obscurity is a loss for the public, most of whom have never heard about these forms of treatment.

As previously mentioned, empiricists are vitalists, that is, they function from the basic premise that there is a vital force, or physis, that is the source of life in all living organisms. This physis is seen as an energy that comes directly from nature and is thought to be responsible for all symptoms and for the healing process itself. Thus, the empiricist considers himself or herself to be subordinate to this flow of nature and must obey its laws. This form of medicine is, therefore, based on age-old principles that have been derived through direct observation of how living beings become ill and how they heal.

Symptoms of disease are considered to be generated by the physis as an attempt to heal the organism and are treated, if treatment is needed at all, by assisting in the healing process. Each disease is seen as an individual case and can only be understood through direct observation of the sick person. Treatment must be individual, a fact that necessarily leads to a vast materia medica, or body of substances used as remedies.

Not only is the individual of utmost importance within empiricist medicine, the symptoms that are characteristic of the patient's individual response to disease are more important to the empiricist physician than are the common symptoms of disease. The emotional and mental state of the individual patient is also important in determining treatment, as are dreams and general characteristics. And successful treatment is evaluated not only by the disappearance of symptoms, but also by the fact that the cure moves the patient in a direction that has been shown to lead to an increase in health and vitality.

In all, the empiricist approach is respectful of nature and open to many possibilities that may present themselves within the framework of its tradition. Training for an empiricist means understanding the laws of nature regarding health and disease and the knowledge of many remedies. It also requires that the physician not allow his or her own prejudices to stand in the way of understanding and observing the individual.

The advantages of empiricist medicine are not only that it alleviates disease but also that it is capable of improving the state of health in general. Treatments are individualized, so there is no problem with remedies becoming useless. Because empiricist medicine treats by stimulating the organisms own healing potential, there is little need for using toxic medicines, and empiricist medicine is effective even when drug-resistant organisms are involved in the disease process.

Empiricist medicine is particularly useful in vague disease states that are difficult to diagnose or when the disease is actually the result of emotional problems such as post-traumatic stress disorder.

The disadvantages of empiricist medicine are usually seen if it is used without addressing symptoms that are mechanical in nature. Problems requiring surgery usually demand a more mechanistic approach and may be better resolved by a rationalist physician. Most of the disadvantages of empiricist medicine are, however, not experienced by the patient but by the physician. With its huge materia medica and need to observe the entirety of each individual case, empiricist medicine demands continual study and close patient contact. It is also extremely time consuming. Because of this, a physician following the empiricist path in medicine must constantly develop his or her skills, spend much time in practice, and see a more limited number of patients than a rationalist physician.

Living with Paradox

After briefly reviewing the division that exists between philosophies of medicine and between rational and symbolic thinking, it becomes obvious that humanity has separated itself from nature. Although this separation was necessary, it may also become clear that the next step is to utilize the opposite poles within that division to construct an entirely new paradigm. To do this, one needs the ability to accept paradox. Indeed it is the ability to accept paradox that is characteristic of this new paradigm of medicine. According to Jung, "only the paradox comes anywhere near to comprehending the fullness of life. Non-ambiguity and non-contradiction are one-sided and thus unsuited to express the incomprehensible."[4]

The physician utilizing the new paradigm of medicine would be asked to understand and respect both empiricism and rationalism. The physician would be unlikely to practice both forms, but should know when it was appropriate to refer to one or the other. Medical schools would require that students relinquish the idea that it is they who cure and understand that they are midwives to the healing process inherent within Mother Nature.

This is not an easy feat—for it has been characteristic of human nature to take a stance and defend it against all intruders. The building of an individual ego separate from the forces of nature has been a hard won struggle, and what is being asked now is to subordinate the ego to the greater good. Fortunately we have within empiricist medicine, and specifically homeopathy, guidelines for health that include development of the whole person. They include developing a mental state of increased clarity of mind and creativity and the ability to use these for the well-being of others, as well as for oneself. Another guideline for health is an increase in the ability for love, respect, happiness, and the ability to be a positive influence on others. These are not purely theoretical ideas; many people who have been treated by homeopathy have realized these goals. Their voices will be heard in this book.

The fact that these guidelines are already in place in a medical system, and that they have been achieved by some, points to the possibility that generosity, compassion, and love are characteristics of healthy human beings and that selfishness, hatred, and lack of concern for the welfare of others, while certainly part of the human condition, are capable of being integrated and healed.

The world of dreams has much to contribute to this new paradigm of medicine. Many people are not aware of the opposites inherent within themselves and remain unconscious of the fact that they are living only one side of the reality of who they are. Dreams compensate for this one-sided view and allow the dreamer to see his shadow side. Integration of the shadow is an essential step in developing a more conscious attitude toward life. By integrating the shadow, one begins to see that he or she contains within what he or she has been projecting onto others.

This realization allows for a broadening of consciousness that renders the individual more capable of seeing other points of view, an awareness that is particularly important to the practitioner of the healing arts. Discrimination between good and evil, right and wrong remain an essential part of life, but it is no longer necessary to identify with those views. This is crucial because much of what has been declared to be a fight for right and wrong has led to schisms, power struggles, and attempts to destroy those philosophies and healing methods that conflict with a particular belief.

Dreams can help to integrate the paradox of opposites existing within the same reality, give messages to compensate for behaviors that are leaning too far in one direction or another, and help practitioners to understand the mind-body relationship. Working with dreams requires that we momentarily leave behind dearly held ideas of reality and immerse ourselves into a realm pregnant with new ideas. It is a creative experience that opens the mind to new possibilities and solutions.

The Dream

A thin young man sits perfectly still in the corner of a pristine white stage. He has two large heads, shiny and black. As he turns toward me, the black masklike faces look faintly familiar, evoking a vague memory of some ancient African shaman. The young man is surrounded by an aura of mystery and power that is awe-inspiring and somewhat frightening. I wake with a start. It was a dream.

I had asked for a dream message to be given to me over a period of three consecutive nights for the purpose of this book. The following night, I found myself staring at this two-headed fellow. He was a complex symbol, strange and familiar, frightening and fascinating.

In an attempt to further understand what this meant and how I was to use it, I began to explore each part of the symbol using the same process of dream analysis that I have engaged in, with the guidance of a Jungian analyst, for almost ten years. This process considers the dreamer's own association to the imagery to be of primary importance and is viewed within the context of the dreamer's life. It also requires that the dreamer's personal association to each and every aspect of the dream image be explored in minute detail.

This time, however, going through my personal associations to the parts of the image was not revealing the meaning. It seemed unrelated to my personal state. The mysterious power of this image suggested the presence of a more universal or archetypal symbol. Archetypal symbols are universal patterns or motifs that are common to humanity in general. They are seen throughout the ages in mythologies, religions, and fairy tales and, as such, are beyond what can be understood through personal associations. Understanding archetypal symbolism in a dream requires research into the meaning of the symbol on a universal level.

For the purpose of discovering this meaning, I began to do some research using the library of books that I had collected over the years for just this purpose. Beginning with an outstanding feature of the symbol, the two heads, I came across many ideas for the number two—the first division of reality, conflict, or the alpha and the omega, the beginning and the end. The idea of the alpha and omega was interesting. After all, this is the beginning of the book, and because it is an overview, it is also the end. This reminded me of the *uroborus*—the circular symbol from alchemy of a dragon or snake biting its own tail, which Jung calls the basic mandala of alchemy. "Time and again," says Jung in *Psychology and Alchemy*, referring to the symbolic meaning of the uroborus, "the alchemists reiterate that the *opus* proceeds from the one and leads back to the one.... Mercurius stands at the beginning and the end of the work: he is the *prima materia*, the *caput corvi*, the *nigredo;* as dragon he devours himself and as dragon he dies, to rise again as the *lapis*."⁵

Going back to my dream symbol, the figure was not simply about the number two—it had two heads. I was, after all, getting quite heady from writing. Was this what the dream was telling me? I felt that there was a deeper meaning.

The heads were black—my association to black or darkness is that it is about the unconscious depths of the psyche—the unknown. Black also refers to alchemical term *nigredo,* the darkness that breaks down matter so transformation may take place.

It suddenly occurred to me that the two-headed image is a hermaphrodite—another alchemical symbol, indicating the two in one and the merging of opposites. This motif appears again and again in alchemy, including in the Rosarium pictures, a series of woodcuts from the fifteenth century. Many feel that the Rosarium pictures are not only the alchemist's portrayal of the transformation process of the chemicals in his flasks, but the transformation of the alchemist himself.

Then it began to come together. The idea of *prima materia,* the hermaphrodite, allusions to the transformation process and even the uroborus—all pointed to that ultimate trickster, Mercurius. Moreover it was not Mercurius in general, but Mercurius as the *filius hermaphroditus.* The filius hermaphroditus is the alchemists' representation of "the water of the philosophers," the substance that transmutes the elements of the substance undergoing the alchemical process, and in transforming the substance becomes transformed.

At this point I understood something of the dream but was still dissatisfied. Fortunately, I had given myself three days of dreaming, so I waited for further clarification.

The following night I couldn't remember any dream. As I thought about the irony of having no dream, I began to recall the two-headed symbol—whereas in the original dream it was sitting passively, it now seemed animated, as if it had taken on more life force. (N.B.: the practice of working with dream material in the waking state is known as active imagination.) Suddenly, I was writing this chapter in my head and had to get out of bed and capture what was writing itself.

I was inspired to write about the dream process as it happened, elucidating the experience of working with dreams and symbols. Thus, the reader would be able to directly experience the archetypal realms of the psyche.

The symbol as Mercurius in the form of the filius hermaphroditus began to make more sense. Here we have an aspect of Mercurius as the underlying force of alchemical transmutation. It is no mere coincidence that Mercury holds in his hand the caduceus that has become the symbol of medicine. The caduceus was originally the magic wand of Aesculapius and had only one snake, signifying that the god heals, but the caduceus of Mercurius contains two snakes, symbolic of the process of *coniunctio,* or combination, that takes place in the alchemist's retort. Jung recounts the story of the alchemist Maier, who, so the story goes, met his mentor, Mercurius. Mercurius handed over his art and wisdom to Maier, along with the magic caduceus, to aid him in his work. Here Jung says, "The sacred snake of the Asklepion signified: The god heals; but the caduceus, or Mercurius in the form of the coniunctio in the retort, means: In the hands of the physician lie the magic remedies granted by God."[6]

Mercurius and the caduceus are symbolic of the archetype of the healer. After this encounter, I felt inspired and in touch with the concepts of healing that comprise much of this book. However, as the day went on, nothing seemed to be going right, and a pervasive feeling of negativity began to color my experience.

The third night of dreaming made the situation even worse. This was supposed to be the pièce de résistance, the dream that brought everything together; but instead I had a dream that I immediately wanted to disregard. In the dream, I was at a party where men and women were dancing and having a lot of fun, but no one asked me to dance. This was especially painful because they were playing the tango, my favorite dance. I felt left out and angrily walked out of the party into a dark rainy night, alone and weeping.

I thought, "This dream couldn't possibly be relevant—I'll just leave it out." I was experiencing resistance to a truth that I didn't want to see.

Dreams often do this—they compensate for what is being experienced in the waking state. In the previous dream, I had an encounter with Mercurius, the archetype of healing. Any experience of the archetypal realm holds a danger—that of identifying with an area that is larger than human, what the ancients called the realm of the gods. This creates an inflation of the ego. The ego thinks that it has the qualities of the numinous symbol.

Looking at all parts of the third dream, I saw that it not only had deep personal significance but was an attempt on the part of my psyche to compensate for that inflation. Dancing, and particularly the tango, represents for me a celebration of the intertwining of opposites, of male and female. In the dream, I am denied this experience and leave the celebration, moving out alone into the darkness. It is the opposite of the combination in the alchemical flask and the union of the two serpents on the magical staff that contains remedies from the gods.

If we look at this series of dreams, we may see it as an encounter with Mercurius as the archetype of the healer in general and more specifically as the alchemical water of the philosophers, the force that transmutes and transforms in the healing process. As the god who moves from heaven to Earth and down into the underworld, Mercurius is not only heaven but also hell. He personifies the ability to move from one opposite to the other. Thus, he represents the healer and the process of healing as a phenomenon that contains a powerful duality.

In *The Alchemy of Healing*, Jungian psychologist and homeopath Edward Whitmont talks about the duality within the archetype of healing:

> *Mankind suffers illness; human beings inflict wounds and hurt each other and themselves. We suffer our own inner conflicts and inflict them on one another, and we help heal one another. We also inflict wounds and injuries upon the physical world we live in. As the destruction and consciousness-carrying "cells" of the earth organism, we wound our earth, we interfere with its vital functioning and, as our consciousness of self and world gradually increases, we also strive to heal these wounds.*
>
> *Wounding, being wounded and healing are functional aspects of one and the same archetypal pattern, of the same autonomous, transpersonal, a priori, in-formational expression of implicate-order entelechy.[7]*

The archetype of healing encompasses not only healing, but being wounded and wounding. This is akin to the homeopathic principle of the law of similars: That which causes a problem can also cure it. Failure to understand this concept leads to identification with only the healing aspect of the archetype. This may result in egotistical and power-driven behavior that harms not only the patient but the practitioner as well. The practitioner becomes possessed by a "god complex" and dominates others in a way that is dangerous to others and to the practitioner. In his book *Power in the Helping Professions*, Jungian analyst Adolf Guggenbühl-Craig tells us that the modern cult surrounding the physician is at least partly an expression of this power.

The symbolic imagery emerging from my dreams points to the filius hermaphroditus as containing both healing, represented by the magical caduceus, and wounding, symbolized by the dream of alienation and isolation. The dreams suggest that both are integral parts of the alchemical transformation necessary in healing and represent, through the symbolism of the water of the philosophers, the healing substance that becomes transformed, the inner capacity for self-healing as well as the external healer. According to Guggenbühl-Craig, there is no special healer archetype or patient archetype.

> *The healer and the patient are two aspects of the same. When a person becomes sick, the healer-patient archetype is constellated. The sick man seeks an external healer, but at the same time the intra-psychic healer is activated. We often refer to this intra-psychic healer in the ill as the "healing factor." It is the physician within the patient himself and its healing action (that) is as great as that of the doctor who appears on the scene externally. Neither wounds nor diseases can heal without the curative action of the inner healer.*[8]

The urge toward healing represented by Mercurius is a deep and instinctual inner drive within the human mind, body, and spirit, and is not limited to the healing profession.

Mercurius and his caduceus are, however, a symbol of the healing profession and the god of alchemy, who was thought to assist the alchemist in his work. The spirit of Mercurius, or Hermes as he was also known, was greatly appreciated by the alchemists as the spirit within all matter, a fact that would also make him very aligned to the art of homeopathy.

According to Jung, alchemical symbolism was a projection of the contents of the alchemist's unconscious onto matter and brought those contents to light. Because this symbolism occurred at a time when very little was known about the unconscious, Jung felt that the images were an untainted projection that could be useful in understanding the nature of the psyche.

> *This was a time when the mind of the alchemist was still grappling with the problems of matter, when the exploring consciousness was confronted by the dark void of the unknown, in which figures and laws were dimly perceived and attributed to matter although they really belonged to the psyche. Everything unknown and empty is filled with psychological projection; it is as if the investigator's own psychic background were mirrored in the darkness. What he sees in matter, or thinks he can see, is chiefly the data of his own unconscious, which he is projecting into it.*[9]

Jung spent much of his later life researching alchemical texts and used alchemical symbols and processes to describe the nature of the psyche and its transformation during the development of the individual personality. The fact that many people today know nothing about alchemy and still have dream images that bear a striking resemblance to the alchemical process validates Jung's theory. Although we no longer see matter in the way in which the alchemists perceived it, our unconscious is still going through its own alchemical process.

Mercurius, one of the most frequently used symbols, represents the transformation that the alchemist himself goes through during his work to distill *prima materia*, or basic matter, into the philosopher's stone. In alchemy, the philosopher's stone is a metaphor for the successful transmutation of base metal into gold. From a psychological point of view, it is an archetypal symbol of wholeness. Mercurius is the lowly beginning of the work as the *prima materia* and also its highest goal, the lapis, or *ultima materia*. Through Mercurius, the alchemist turned lead into gold. Therefore, Mercurius plays a large part in the inner alchemy of the unconscious and may be seen as an essential part of the healing process.

Nevertheless, Mercurius is also a trickster and a very wily fellow. He runs all over the place, from heaven to hell. As much as he is light, he is also darkness. Many-sided, changeable, and deceitful, he drove the alchemist to despair. Therefore, the wise alchemist knew better than to allow Mercurius to run free in the initial phases of the alchemical process. The alchemist kept Mercurius safely closed in a clear glass flask, sealed with the sign of Hermes. (Thus the derivation of the phrase "hermetically sealed.") There he remained until the alchemical distillation was complete and he was transformed into the lapis.

The two-headed figure in my dream represents the dual-natured Mercurius as the spirit of healing, wild and unrefined. He is the vital principle, flowing naturally in an instinctive, naive, and unconscious way. In order to guide the spirit of healing, the practitioner must use conscious awareness to bottle Mercurius up so transformation can occur. Thus the practitioner's awareness of the healing process serves as an alchemical flask in which the dual nature of mind and body, and opposing forces characteristic of the derangement of the vital principle, are integrated into psychosomatic balance.

Placing Mercurius in the bottle creates an environment in which the natural tendency toward healing can be guided by the practitioner and lessens Mercurius's wild tendencies. He does, however, still maintain some of his tricks, one of which is that he ultimately changes those who work with him. If the work is done consciously and the bottle remains sealed until the end, the change is for good. If the work is not done consciously, the practitioner can take on some of the grandiosity, darkness, or other of the negative aspects within the dual nature of this wily god.

The following chapters of this book are meant to serve as a guide for understanding the relationship between the healing process and the transformation of the psyche, and to give the homeopath and others interested in healing, a method to implement this healing process. As such, it is a guide to building one's own alchemical flask in which to distill the spirit of Mercurius.

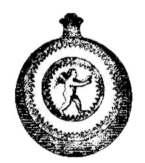

Mercurius in the vessel, Barchusen,
Elementa Chemiae (1718)

CHAPTER TWO

Homeopathy
Mind-Body Medicine

Homeopathy is an empirical system of medicine that uses nontoxic remedies to stimulate the inherent healing capacity within the mind and body. It was founded by Samuel Hahnemann, a German physician who, more than two hundred years ago, not only created a radically new form of therapy in homeopathy but formulated a scientific system to understand health, disease, and healing on a fundamental level. In his *Organon of the Medical Art*, a text still studied by homeopaths, he summarized the results of his research into subjects such as diathesis, or inherited tendencies in disease; the role of the mind in medical treatment; and the compassionate treatment of mental illness. He also explored the relationship between acute and chronic manifestations and gave instructions for the treatment of epidemic disease.

Hahnemann's theories about the treatment of epidemic disease were put to the test during the typhoid, cholera, and scarlet fever epidemics in Europe in the mid and late 1800s. Patients under homeopathic treatment had a much better survival rate than those under any other form of treatment. In the southern United States, homeopathy again showed its effectiveness in the yellow fever epidemic of 1876. People treated with standard allopathic treatment had at least a 16 percent mortality rate, while the mortality rate of those treated with homeopathy was 7.7 percent.[1]

Born in 1755, Hahnemann lived and practiced at the time of heroic medicine, when physicians, if they were not busy bleeding their patients, were poisoning them with large amounts of mercury and arsenic. The population who visited doctors was rendered severely ill from the toxic and depleting treatments that frequently caused more harm than good. Abhorring this type of treatment and realizing that it was not helping to cure disease, Hahnemann left his medical practice and became a translator of medical texts.

While translating a text by William Cullen on the treatment of malaria with Peruvian bark, Hahnemann came across a statement that caught his attention. Cullen wrote that Peruvian bark, or *China officinalis,* cured malaria because it was a bitter and astringent herb. Hahnemann felt that, if this were true, other bitter and astringent herbs should work as well, and he knew that they didn't. In the true investigative spirit of the scientist he was, Hahnemann conducted an experiment on himself. He ingested Peruvian bark repeatedly for many days and documented the resulting symptoms: chills, sweats, and intermittent fever, the symptoms of malaria. His experiment proved that Peruvian bark cured the symptoms of malaria because it had within it the capacity to cause the symptoms of this disease in a healthy person. In addition, he developed a method through which the law of similars, a principle of healing long understood by ancient physicians, could be more accurately applied.

The Law of Similars

Long before Hahnemann founded homeopathy, the law of similars was a known principle by which physicians could apply different therapies. Hippocrates mentioned cure by similars, and Paracelsus, a sixteenth-century German physician and alchemist, wrote that all treatment should be based on the principle of similars. The basic premise is: that a substance that can cause a symptom can also cure it. An example of the law of similars in conventional medicine is the use of immunizations and allergy treatments. In these cases, a small amount of the pathogen or allergen is given to stimulate the immune response. Although these treatments are examples of the principle of cure by similars, it must be noted that these treatments are not based on other homeopathic principles, such as the need for individualized treatment and the unique method of preparation of homeopathic remedies.

Psychotherapists have also used the principle of similars. Jungian psychologists are aware that, for healing to occur, there must be some similarity between the personality and psychological terrain of the analyst and analysand. If they are not similar enough, it is unlikely that the analysand will be able to make the deep and intimate connection to the therapist that is required for a successful analysis.

In general, therapies based on the principle of similars stimulate the healing process, and therapies based on the application of opposites alleviate but suppress symptoms, sometimes driving the disease to a deeper level. An example of a suppressive treatment is the treatment of childhood eczema with steroids. In many cases, although the skin problem disappears, the child may end up with asthma.

Application of the law of opposites requires extensive diagnosis to recognize a myriad of diseases that are then treated with relatively few general medicines. Healing techniques that utilize similars require many more medicines and match them not to the disease but to the individual.

The application of the law of similars is an essential part of understanding homeopathy, and the cultivation of the ability to apply this law is an ongoing development in the practice of homeopathy. It requires the homeopath to perceive the unique combination of symptoms in an individual and match that symptom complex to a remedy known to cause that particular pattern of symptoms. If the remedy is not a close enough match, it will do nothing. If the match is close or exact, the remedy will resonate with the individual and will stimulate a process of healing.

One can better understand the need for resonance by looking at a process that has begun to be better understood by neuroscientists over the last years: the relationship between receptors in a cell and chemicals called ligands. Each cell in the body is covered with receptors that act as sensing agents and have the ability to pick up ligands affecting the function of the cell. Ligands can be neurotransmitters such as norepinephrine or peptides that act as neurotransmitters or steroids like cortisol. These chemicals cause complex and fundamental changes in the cells onto whose receptors they lock.

What is relevant to the law of similars is that these receptors only respond to a chemical that fits the receptor, as a key fits into a lock. A more accurate way of explaining this is that the receptor only responds when a particular chemical has enough resonance with it to stimulate a response, a reaction that could be compared with the bodily changes that go on when the "chemistry" is right between two people on a first date. When this cell "chemistry" is right, the chemical from outside of the cell is let into the interior of the cell creating deep changes within the cell matter. Likewise, the correct homeopathic remedy is somehow able to resonate with the body and mind in such a way that it stimulates deep and profound healing. Perhaps it is functioning as a ligand that is very specific to the individual and resonates with the receptors of the myriad cells of the body.

Provings

Although Hahnemann did not discover the law of similars, his great contribution to its applications was a means to apply this law of healing systematically. He developed a method to discover symptoms that particular medicines could cause and therefore cure. This technique, called proving a remedy, led to the creation of a scientifically verified materia medica that could be used by anyone trained in the practice of homeopathy. This materia medica currently fills a vast number of books, listing the origin, application, and dosage of approximately 3,000 homeopathic remedies. Before provings, only individuals with a deep intuitive sense could understand how medicinal substances would affect the whole person, on the mental and emotional as well as the physical level, and apply these substances according to known principles of healing.

Information on how the remedies are to be used comes from provings like the experiments Hahnemann conducted, as well as from accidental provings or poisonings and clinical data from cured symptoms.

Provings are a form of research that is conducted using healthy human beings, something that is possible because the remedies are diluted until they are nontoxic. A group of people, usually homeopaths and homeopathic students, volunteer to take a homeopathic remedy, and their reaction is closely supervised. The study is now conducted in a double-blind test, meaning neither the prover nor the supervisor is aware of the substance being proved. The provers write down all of the symptoms they experience that are different from their usual physical, emotional, and mental state in a journal. At the end of the proving, which may last anywhere from a one to six months or more, the symptoms of all of the provers are collected and organized.

The results of the proving are then published, usually in homeopathic journals. If the remedy has been shown to be one that may be useful, it enters into the homeopathic materia medica. The ultimate result of a useful proving is a pattern of symptoms or characteristic qualities unique to the substance and applicable to the clinical practice of homeopathy.

Another discovery made by Hahnemann during his provings of the original two hundred or so remedies he tested, was the relationship between mental and emotional symptoms. He saw that when people developed symptoms during a proving, those symptoms were not only physical but also mental. Thus he deduced that, when an individual gets ill, the mind as well as the body exhibits symptoms, and the remedy that will cure the illness needs to address the whole person and the totality of their disease.

Micro Dilutions

Hahnemann first proved substances in measurable physical amounts, primarily as herbal tinctures and minerals. Because he was able to utilize them in a more exact way than earlier physicians who applied the principle of similars, he achieved very good result in the treatment of disease. However, he now ran into a dilemma. He knew from his experiments that substances could cure the symptoms they caused in healthy persons, but he also realized that many medicines were poisons that had the capacity to cause severe problems and even death.

After much thought, he decided to try diluting a poison to the level at which it would be nontoxic. Unfortunately, the resulting remedy was totally ineffective. Being the avid experimenter that he was, he went back to the drawing board and tried another way of diluting it. This time he succussed, or vigorously shook, the poison in between each successive dilution. Through this process of dilution and succussion, he succeeded in making a remedy that was both nontoxic and had healing properties. To the present day, homeopathic remedies are made through this process of dilution and succussion.

The use of highly dilute remedies has been one of the most controversial aspects of homeopathy. Most remedies are diluted beyond the point at which there is any probability of any molecule of the original substance is left. This fact has brought forth cries of outrage from the scientific community, with accusations of "it's a placebo" and "there's nothing in it, so it must be a fraud." According to Dana Ullman, internationally recognized educator on homeopathic medicine, people who insist that homeopathy is quackery because the remedies are so dilute are themselves being unscientific. "It is as though they are saying," he writes in *The Consumer's Guide to Homeopathy*,[2] "that these medicines can't work because they don't fit our present paradigm of medicine and physics. These people are usually unfamiliar with the controlled studies or the wide body of clinical experience with homeopathic medicine in the homeopathic and conventional literature." For up-to-date information on research and studies on homeopathy, refer to Dana Ullman's e-book, *Homeopathic Family Medicine*.[3]

Although there are still many who doubt, research has shown that when substances are diluted and succussed to the level used in homeopathy they have the same effect on the receptors of the cell as the gross substance. Drs. Bellavite and Signorini, in *The Emerging Science of Homeopathy: Complexity, Biodynamics, and Nanopharmacology*, cite several research projects on the use of highly diluted substances prepared in a way similar to the preparation of homeopathic remedies. According to them, "A pharmacologically active substance when tested in a highly diluted solution appears to react specifically to the same biological system to which the non-diluted substance reacts."[4]

The Practice of Homeopathy

The homeopath's task is to perceive what needs to be healed in the individual and to match that to a remedy shown to be able to cure that problem. Unlike in conventional medicine, what needs to be healed is not a disease with a name, but rather a repeating pattern of dysfunction that may lead to a disease, disorder, or other type of suffering on the mental, emotional, or physical level. To the untrained eye, the information given in an initial interview with a patient may appear confused or chaotic, particularly because the homeopath gathers information about the entire person, including the patient's general and emotional state, likes and dislikes, dreams and family history, and physical complaints.

The homeopath must view the confused or chaotic state within the individual from a broader and broader perspective until the order reveals itself. Physicist David Bohm tells us that when scientists describe the behavior of a natural system as random, this label may not describe the natural system at all, but rather the observer's degree of understanding of that system—which could be complete ignorance.

This describes what is happening when the physician does not yet understand the order within the individual—all of the symptoms appear as random. Conventional medicine attempts to order this by diagnosis, though a patient inevitably experiences other "extraneous" symptoms that do not fit within a specific diagnosis. In other words, the conventional approach is to categorize a disease by matching a few of the most outstanding symptoms exhibited by the patient to the known symptoms associated with a particular disease. Although this is successful and useful to some extent, in terms of understanding the underlying order or process of the disease it is actually overlaying a previously known, and often inaccurate, reality on the situation.

In contrast, the homeopath, although not negligent of conventional diagnosis, takes the diagnosis to be a useful but small perspective on the actual situation. The homeopath attempts to view the case from a large perspective and unprejudiced outlook so that what first appears to be random is eventually seen as an orderly pattern. If successful in analyzing a case, the homeopath begins to perceive a pattern that repeats itself in every symptom and every aspect of the individual. This is the pattern of what needs to be healed, and when matched to a remedy with a similar pattern, the remedy stimulates the body and mind to heal itself naturally.

Where there is a disease process that can be easily identified and treated through conventional measures, it may be difficult for someone unfamiliar with homeopathy to perceive the difference between the homeopathic and conventional approach. However, when we are confronted by a condition such as CFS, candidiasis, or autoimmune diseases, which typically are syndromes with variable and random symptoms, the difference becomes clear. Even without a complex of symptoms that clearly fit a known disease, it is possible for the homeopath to perceive the order within the case and prescribe an appropriate remedy. This is possible because the symptoms of the whole person, his or her life situation, inheritance, dreams and inclinations, as well as the pathological symptoms are used to find the remedy.

In addition, the homeopath does not attempt to understand the imbalance, syndrome, disease or whatever it may be called in conventional terms. This would create the same situation—that of overlaying or insinuating a preconceived idea or form upon what cannot truly be known. Instead, the homeopath attempts to match the repeating pattern that is the essential order of the individual to a homeopathically prepared substance that has a similar pattern.

Following the Path to Cure

Homeopaths view symptoms as an attempt on the part of the body to heal; therefore, a cure must address the underlying cause of disease, or the general health will suffer. Because the goal is cure, the homeopathic physician is trained to determine if the healing process is going in the right direction. This is vital, because any form of treatment can suppress or palliate symptoms, that is, remove them without healing the underlying cause of disease.

In some cases, suppression of symptoms can cause the actual disease to become even more severe. An example of this is the treatment of fever with aspirin. Fever is an effective way of fighting off disease, and when the fever is suppressed, the body may have more difficulty throwing off the disease. Over 90 percent of children who developed Reye's syndrome, a serious neurological disease, had previously received aspirin to treat the symptoms of flu or another viral disease. It is also possible to suppress emotional symptoms, and psychologists warn of the suffering, conflict and even physical disease caused by this suppression.

On the other hand, suppression of symptoms is sometimes a life-saving measure in emotional as well as physical illness. Therefore, practitioners must know when suppression is necessary and when it may be harmful and to be able to differentiate between suppression, cure, and palliation.

While homeopathic treatment of acute diseases such as colds, flu, and minor injuries must also include knowing the difference between suppression, palliation, and cure, acute homeopathic treatment can be learned quite easily. Persons who are willing to do a bit of studying can learn to treat themselves and their families for minor and self-limiting diseases by taking a short course or studying several of the many books available.

Treatment of chronic disease must, however, be done by a professional homeopath trained in the art and science of homeopathy. In these cases, following the direction of cure becomes much more complicated and takes many years of training to understand. This is especially complicated because the homeopath must consider how the person is doing as a whole, including symptoms on the mental, emotional, and physical level.

Homeopathic philosophy considers symptoms on the mental level, such as disorientation, confusion, and psychosis, to be the deepest level; while emotional symptoms such as anxiety and phobias are considered to be less serious. Physical symptoms are the most superficial. Homeopathy also considers the intensity of the symptom and the degree to which it limits the freedom of the individual. Therefore, a person may have mental or emotional symptoms that are very mild and do not limit his or her life while the physical symptoms are extremely limiting. In such cases, the physical disease would be considered to be the deepest symptom in the individual. For a more detailed view of levels of disease from a homeopathic perspective see *The Science of Homeopathy*, by George Vithoulkas.[5]

The life of theoretical physicist Stephen Hawking illustrates the great importance of mental and emotional health and how that can transcend some of the most difficult physical disabilities. Dr. Hawking, who is almost totally paralyzed, confined to a wheelchair, and must speak through a voice synthesizer because of a neurological disease, has not allowed this to hamper his life. He lectures widely and has written many books on the nature of the universe. On his Web site, he writes the following about his disability:

> *I am quite often asked: How do you feel about having ALS? The answer is, not a lot. I try to lead as normal a life as possible, and not*

think about my condition, or regret the things it prevents me from doing,
which are not that many.[6]

Health and the healing process are more complex than can be evaluated from one perspective, and other methods are also used to determine the direction of cure. One guideline is from an early American homeopath, Constantine Hering, M.D., who observed that there are three directions in which cure proceeds. Hering said that cure proceeds from the most vital to the least vital function, from the top of the body to the bottom, and that the most recent symptoms would disappear before the oldest symptoms.

Hering's law serves as a guideline for the homeopath to evaluate the direction of cure by observing if the disease is becoming more superficial and less restricting to the individual. The homeopath will look for signs of symptoms that endanger the health and freedom of the individual disappearing first and more superficial symptoms that have less impact on life leaving later in the healing process. It is as if the homeopathic healing, led by Mother Nature herself, tries to rid the person of symptoms that are most debilitating and most threatening to a person's survival first.

Another process that is often seen in all of natural healing, including homeopathy, is the retracting of symptoms. This means that a person undergoing the healing process may remember or experience past symptoms in order to give the body and mind an opportunity to heal them.

As a person heals, the homeopath evaluates the improvement taking place in the mental and emotional state of the individual, as well as the improvement in the physical symptoms. Increased energy, better sleep, greater clarity of mind, and an increased ability to experience love are most often a sign that cure is proceeding in the right direction.

Homeopathic treatment stimulates the inherent ability of the mind and body to heal itself naturally. This healing improves the overall health of the person, enabling a fuller and happier life. Each individual who chooses to heal in this way plays a role in improving the quality of life for everyone.

Therapies like homeopathy, which are capable of helping people achieve a greater level of health on the mental and emotional level, as well as alleviating the disease and suffering of the physical body, make an important contribution to the well-being of society for many generations. When the practitioner also understands something of the complexity of the human psyche, these therapies have an even greater possibility of meeting the challenges that are presented by these difficult times.

CHAPTER THREE

Psyche and Soma

Exploring the Mystery of the Mind-Body Relationship

People involved in contemporary medicine show a good deal of interest in the connection between the mind and its role in creating and healing physical disease. However, much of the research into this area is not about the relationship between the mind and the body but rather the brain and the body. The mind itself remains an enigma, and the exploration of such concepts as soul and spirit are, for the most part, relegated to the realm of metaphysics, a field thought by mainstream medicine to be unworthy of science. Science as it is widely practiced today does have an underlying metaphysical belief system, that of scientific realism. This belief is that physical theories represent an independent and objective reality and that laws of nature are revealed using mathematical analysis and empirical verification. This is the unconscious belief of most contemporary scientists, even though many philosophers of science presently reject the idea that scientific theories represent the universe, as it is, independent of our experience.[1]

Because of the influence of scientific realism, even the practice of psychiatry and psychology, which propose to deal with the mind, often develop theories of mental and emotional disease based on chemical imbalances or behavioral problems. Thus, even psychologists may end up practicing the medicine of the psyche as if the psyche doesn't exist.

Scientific realism affects all areas of science and limits the way we perceive ourselves as human beings. For the practitioner of the healing arts, it creates a fundamental dilemma. If the relationship between the mind and body is purely mechanistic and the mind is simply the brain, how then do we explain factors such as someone experiencing chest pains when, unbeknownst to that person, a loved one is having a heart attack? How does one deal with the fact that there are presently over 150 scientific studies showing that prayers, thoughts, and wishes have an affect on distant biological systems, including plants, animals, human beings and microorganisms?[2] Moreover, if the healing process also requires an integration of the spirit and soul, how do we reconcile this with conventional ideas about health and disease?

Even practitioners of homeopathy and other forms of whole body medicine are powerfully affected by this worldview. Many times, what has come to be called complementary medicine is actually a debasement of the underlying philosophies within holistic modalities in order that they may fit more comfortably into the paradigm of conventional medicine. This strategy may allow a temporary gain in acceptance, but it is not, in the long run, in the interest of improved medical care.

What is needed is a model that would allow practitioners of holistic medicine in general, and homeopathy specifically, to work with the mind-body without diluting the underlying philosophy and metaphysics of their healing modality. This is not to say, as many critics of the holistic model maintain, that the conventional, mechanistic model would be disregarded. Rather, it would mean seeing that conventional medicine has its place and appreciating the difference between the underlying belief systems.

Working with the mind-body requires a model that is flexible and able to accept that the mind-body relationship is to some extent measurable, being reflected in the brain, nervous system, and chemistry of the body, and at the same time an immeasurable mystery. An effective model must therefore include a method for the practitioner to develop direct knowledge of the workings of his or her own mind-body.

It would also require a map of the mind-body that allows for the fact that parts of this puzzle will remain unknown and possibly enter into the realm of a form of metaphysics drastically different from scientific realism. It would be understood that this map is not the "territory," and under no circumstances should it become a template in which to categorize patients. The final requirement would be a method of therapeutics that addresses the whole person. This therapy should be philosophically consistent with the idea that the healing process may or may not require integrating the soul and spirit.

I would like to propose a model that would improve the practitioner's ability to understand the mind-body relationship, enabling the practitioner to be more effective in finding the appropriate treatment and following the healing process. This model is drawn from Jung's concept of the psyche and his teaching on the patient-therapist relationship. Although this model could possibly be used with other holistic modalities, for the purpose of this book we will cover its use within the practice of homeopathy.

Development of the Practitioner

Jungian analysts are required to go through their own training analysis before working with others. While this is an excellent way for any therapist to develop, there are other methods of personal growth that are also extremely useful. Whether in analysis or not, one of the primary ways that a practitioner can become more receptive to the workings of his or her own psyche is by journaling and interpreting dreams. This practice is covered in chapter 8 of this book. Meditation and the study of mythology, shamanism, and alchemy are a few of the many methods that may also be useful. The study or practice of one or more of these may be helpful, depending on the practitioner's personal preferences and inclinations. These practices familiarize the practitioner with the symbolic language of the psyche and also serve to make the practitioner aware of other worldviews. This is particularly important because we are living in a society in which the belief in scientific realism serves as the unconscious metaphysical ground affecting almost every aspect of life.

When unconscious belief systems are made conscious, it is easier to be more flexible; thereby recognizing the most effective method of treatment. For instance, the conventional medical approach may be the very best way to deal with a broken arm or ruptured appendix. Here, the concepts belonging to scientific realism and the mechanistic approach to medicine hold true. In the case of soul loss, a more common problem than most conventionally thinking practitioners would guess, an entirely different model, perhaps shamanism, would be more appropriate, since that belief system includes the concept of soul loss. If there is a disorder that has developed since an emotional loss, the best choice of treatment might be homeopathy, because it has a model for working with diseases that come on after an emotional stress.

Currently, patients are referred to other forms of therapy only after conventional medicine or psychotherapy has failed. Practitioners who are more aware of the fundamental differences between conventional and nonconventional systems of medicine would be more able to accurately refer patients to the appropriate modality. Thus, even if a practitioner chooses to hold onto one particular belief system, developing an understanding of the underlying belief systems of other forms of treatment makes the practitioner more flexible.

Many meditation techniques from various religions and areas of the world have the capacity to develop strength and calmness of mind. If practiced regularly, they have a profound effect on the individual. In his book *Gathering the Light: A Psychology of Meditation*, Jungian analyst V. Walter Odajnyk explains the effect of meditation on the psyche. After describing the results of a Rorschach inkblot test on practitioners of meditation, including a masters group of very experienced meditators, Dr. Odajnyk concludes that this experiment is "empirical evidence of the fundamental changes that take place in the cognitive and perceptual operations of the psyche as a result of meditation." He concludes his analysis by describing these changes. "The final characteristic of changes a meditator undergoes is the ending of unconscious projection and of the associative, cognitive, and emotional attachments to the projected forms. Meditation breaks down the projected images, makes one aware of the process of projection, dissolves the images to their original energetic source, and frees one from a blind attachment to what we consider to be 'reality.'"[3]

The practice of meditation is a valuable tool for the practitioner of the healing arts. Meditation increases the ability to see what is actually happening, rather than being blinded by the projection of one's internal state onto the patient. It also increases awareness of the process of projection, giving the meditator greater freedom of choice.

A Model of the Mind-Body

In order for a method of working with the mind-body to be useful, it must be flexible enough to include the physical brain, nervous system, and body chemistry, as well as areas of the mind-body relationship that are not measurable. Jung spent most of his lifetime studying the manifestations of the psyche in his clinical practice of psychiatry and through the study of dreams, mythology, and symbols. He traveled widely, observing the rituals and attitudes of various indigenous cultures and listening to their dreams. From these experiences, he felt that the psyche existed in a spectrum from spiritual to somatic and that it was a physical as well as a mental phenomenon that could not be studied by dividing it into parts. In other words, the term *psyche,* as used by Jung, encompasses the mind, spirit, soul, and body and exists as an indivisible entity.

His method for interpreting the psyche is through symbols that are sometimes expressed through bodily symptoms but are more often seen in the symbolic imagery of dreams. Dreams are thought to contain objective facts that are only misunderstood when the dreamer cannot comprehend their meaning. In any case, these symbols frequently point to a greater reality than can be understood by their literal content.

Jung's attitude toward the observation of the patient was very similar to that of Samuel Hahnemann, the founder of homeopathy. Hahnemann's approach was to be the "unprejudiced observer" of the patient, and Jung's approach was to use symbols found in dreams and bodily symptoms as "expressing an as yet unknown and incomprehensible fact of a mystical nature." He also addressed the dangers of projecting one's own ideas onto the patient and having a preconceived idea of how the patient "should be."

Even though Jung developed a comprehensive theory of the psyche, including the concepts of the personal and collective unconscious, archetypes, and the shadow, he approached each person as an individual and judiciously refrained from fitting his patients into that model. His ability to suspend judgment and allow healing to proceed is seen in the following case, recorded in *The Practice of Psychotherapy*.

A young woman, who had been unsuccessfully treated by two other therapists, had a series of bizarre dreams, including one in which a white elephant was coming out of her genitals. The dreams were followed by a series of very intense physical symptoms, the cause of which could not be determined by her physician. She developed uterine ulcers, which finally disappeared but were followed by irritation of the bladder and frequent urination. Since no infection in the bladder could be found, Jung felt the symptoms were symbolic of the young woman's need to express herself and suggested she begin a series of drawings. She drew brightly colored, symmetrical flowers, and the bladder symptoms disappeared, but she soon developed intestinal spasms and explosive diarrhea. These spasms moved up the body until she finally developed a strange feeling, as if her skull were growing soft and a large bird was piercing the top of her head.

At this point, Jung became very concerned and told the patient that he could do nothing more for her. She answered in amazement, "But it's going splendidly! It doesn't matter that you don't understand my dreams. I always have the craziest symptoms, but something is happening all the time."

Even though Jung could not understand her neurosis, he took her at her word and continued to work with her. Around the time that the patient was experiencing the symptoms in her skull, Jung came across a book on Kundalini Yoga that described the raising of spiritual energy in the yogi. The symptoms were almost exactly what his patient had experienced. After learning this, he was able to use the symbolism from this Eastern spiritual system to help her integrate her experiences. Although the patient ended up in a healthy state, Jung concluded that this case was not a "story of triumph." It was "more like a saga of blunders, hesitations, doubts, gropings in the dark, and false clues which in the end took a favorable turn."

After he presented this case, Jung wrote that the psyche must be approached with an open mind, even if what is happening is confusing to the therapist.

> *No psychotherapist should lack that natural reserve which prevents people from riding roughshod over mysteries they do not understand and trampling them flat. This reserve will enable him to pull back in good time when he encounters the mystery of the patient's difference from himself, and to avoid the danger—unfortunately too real—of committing psychic murder in the name of therapy.*[4]

This case is a testament not only to Jung's ability to remain the unprejudiced observer in the difficult process of psychoanalysis; it is a valuable model for how to address the mind-body question. It demonstrates the importance of remaining open to the unknown while utilizing conventional medicine. Moreover, it warns of the "psychic murder" that can so easily take place if the mystery of the individual's healing path is disregarded and an attempt is made to fit the patient into a predetermined view of the reality of health and disease.

Methods of Therapeutics

Working with the mind-body relationship requires a method of treatment that addresses the whole person and is philosophically consistent with the idea that the healing process may require integrating the human soul, spirit, and mind. At the same time, no attempt should be made to rigidly define what is meant by soul, spirit, and mind, as these ideas are essentially unknowable.

In paragraph nine of his *Organon of the Medical Art*, Samuel Hahnemann expresses his view of the relationship between mind, body, and spirit while refraining from defining them:

> *In the healthy human state, the spirit-like life force (autocracy) that enlivens the material organism as dynamis, governs without restriction and keeps all parts of the organism in admirable, harmonious, vital operation, as regards both feelings and functions, so that our indwelling, rational spirit can freely avail itself of this living, healthy instrument for the higher purposes of our existence.*[5]

Homeopathy is a method of therapeutics that is extremely useful in this regard, because it is prescribed on an observation of the physical, emotional, and mental symptoms of the patient, not on a theory regarding the relationship of the body and mind. While the homeopath may use conventional diagnosis as a guide, it is the patient's experience, along with what can be observed, that are of utmost consideration in finding the correct remedy.

The homeopath does not categorize the patient's experience; he or she attempts to perceive what needs to be healed from a fresh perspective. Once this has been perceived, the pattern of the patient's symptoms is matched to the simillimum, or remedy, that has the capability of curing that pattern of symptoms. In his book *Psyche and Substance*, homeopath and Jungian analyst Edward Whitmont describes the elegance of the possibility of healing by giving a substance from nature to heal a similar pattern of disease:

> *It is an amazing testimony to the unity of cosmic existence that the analogous dynamic is also to be found on the biological and organic level in temperamental, constitutional and "acute" adaptive imbalances in the form of illnesses which call for their archetypal counterpattern to be confronted through the simillimum in its attenuated "symbolic" potency or dynamic essence.*[6]

The simillimum allows for the unique expression of the essence of the individual, the possibility that physical disease may or may not be connected with the emotional and mental state of the individual, and does not require a theory as to the relationship between the mind and body.

Homeopathic philosophy sees all symptoms, whether physical, emotional, or mental as the best attempt on the part of the organism to heal itself. Thus the homeopath works to find a remedy that will stimulate this natural healing capacity.

Homeopaths recognize that emotional trauma can also be stored in the body as pain or tension and that it is not unusual for a person to experience memory of trauma as the body heals. Conversely, homeopathy recognizes that symptoms in the body can reappear as the emotional state improves.

A dramatic case that illustrates this is that of a young woman, Giselle, who was treated with homeopathy for poor self-image and periods of severe depression. In her childhood, Giselle had been severely abused mentally and was brutally beaten by her mother. After receiving the homeopathic remedy *Stramonium,* her mental outlook and emotional state improved. In the first month of her treatment black and blue marks appeared over parts of her body where, more than twenty years before, she had been beaten by her mother. The bruises lasted for a few weeks and then disappeared.

Both homeopathy and Jungian psychology are powerful healing modalities on their own. Both address the mind-body relationship, approach the patient from a nonjudgmental perspective, and are concerned with individualized treatment. While homeopathy focuses more on the selection and action of an indicated remedy, both entail a large amount of intense interaction between the patient and practitioner.

In cases where the homeopathic remedy is difficult to find because the indicating symptoms are physically suppressed by medications or other therapies or because the cause of the illness lies deep within the unconscious for unknown reasons, the knowledge of the psyche and its dreams and symbols given to us by Jung is an invaluable addition to the practice of homeopathy. In addition, the wealth of knowledge about the healing relationship between practitioner and patient in Jungian psychology has the capacity to enhance the homeopathic interview and enable the homeopath to be more effective in eliciting symptoms during the initial interview and to follow the healing process. Finally, the process of the homeopath connecting with his psyche, borrowed from the Jungian tradition of the teaching analysis, broadens and clarifies the perception of the homeopath, allowing the practitioner to discriminate between the contents of his or her own psyche and that of the patient, resulting in a more accurate perception of what needs to be healed.

PART II

The Mercurial Fountain
The Inner World of the Psyche

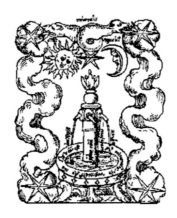

The Mercurial fountain, also known as the mandala fountain, is an image used by the alchemists to portray the chaos from which everything emerges. It represents wholeness, all of the opposites of reality. Everything is there that is needed for transformation to occur, but in a still unrealized state. As such, the image represents the entire contents of the psyche, parts of which must be understood and made conscious during the healing process. In order to effectively utilize dreams in homeopathic practice, it is first necessary to look into the nature of these parts of the psyche, or archetypes.

This next section will explore the nature of the psyche as defined by psychologist Carl Jung. He described the psyche as the totality of all psychological processes, unconscious as well as conscious. Through a lifetime of observing patients, he discovered that, although the psyche manifests itself in many ways depending on the individual, there are qualities to the psyche that could be defined. Unlike Freud, he observed that there is a collective as well as a personal aspect to the unconscious, and this collective unconscious is made up of psychic predispositions inherited by all human beings. He named these ancestral predispositions archetypes and found that, although there were seemingly unlimited numbers of them, some were met again and again in clinical practice. These were, according to Jung, the shadow, the anima and animus, and the Self.

CHAPTER FOUR

Archetypes and the Collective Unconscious

The mind has grown to its present state of consciousness as an acorn grows into an oak or as saurians developed into mammals. As it has for so long been developing, so it still develops, and thus we are moved by forces from within as well as by stimuli from without.

C. G. JUNG, *MAN AND HIS SYMBOLS*[1]

Knowledge of the collective unconscious is essential in order to use the symbolic content of dreams and visions in a fruitful way. Without this knowledge, the symbolism lacks its true meaning and appears simply as a way to deal with the immediate stresses of everyday life. This results in indifference to the guidance available from the vast reservoir of wisdom and intelligence contained within the collective unconscious.

In order to help facilitate the therapeutic use of dreams and symbols, we will first look at the difference between the personal and the collective unconscious and then explore symbols and their role in communication between the former and the latter. We will then examine the nature of archetypes and archetypal symbolism and attempt to understand how they relate to the healing process.

In the Western world, when most people consider the unconscious, they think of Sigmund Freud. Freud's theory is that the unconscious is made up of an individual's repressed and forgotten memories, thoughts, and feelings. The unconscious also includes impulses that have been subliminally registered, like scenes viewed in our peripheral vision. Jung agreed with Freud's definition of the unconscious but felt that it was limited, covering only the personal unconscious. According to Jung, material from the personal unconscious is filled with personal stories and long-forgotten memories, but he also believed the unconscious had another dimension.

Through observation of disturbed individuals, he saw that the contents of their dreams and fantasies could not be limited to their personal experience. He perceived that these individuals had entered into a realm of ancient symbolism to which they had no conscious access. Their dreams and fantasies often contained mythological themes that existed in cultures they had never visited and times previous to the birth of any of their relatives. From these observations, he developed his theory of the collective unconscious, which he defined as the ancestral heritage of possibilities of representation common to all human beings and, perhaps, even all animals.[2]

Because Jung wished to understand complicated psychological conditions and be able to speak about them, he developed a language to express the facts that he observed. He called themes that emerged from the timeless realms of the collective unconscious archetypes. Archetypes, he said, were what made up the contents of the collective unconscious and had a powerful effect on the individual. The discovery of the collective unconscious and the theory of the archetypes are two of Jung's major contributions to psychology.

Because he developed a way to express the functioning of the psyche, Jung has had a very large and many times unacknowledged influence on language in contemporary society. Commonly used terms such as *introvert, extravert, complex, anima, animus, synchronicity,* and *archetypes* are Jungian concepts that are well known but often misused. Because of the misunderstanding of Jung's language, his work is sometimes dismissed as metaphysical. In reality, Jung was a psychiatrist who was able to help some of the most deeply disturbed psychiatric patients through his ability to be the "unprejudiced observer" of their psychic reality. He developed ways of speaking about what was completely within the bounds of human experience, yet he had the uncanny ability to accept even the wildest fantasies of psychotic patients as a valid expression of their reality. Jung would take even the most bizarre flights of fancy very seriously, for he understood that there was a deeper meaning behind these expressions of the psyche and would accept them as a necessary manifestation of the individual's dilemma.

One of his most famous cases is known as "the woman who lived on the moon." When Marie-Louise von Franz, who eventually became one of his closest colleagues, first met Jung, he told her that he was working with a woman who lived on the moon. Von Franz thought that he meant the woman *thought* she lived on the moon. Jung made it clear that the woman lived on the moon. This subtle but important distinction is a major difference between the Jungian approach and most other schools of psychology. Jung's premise was that it was necessary to be completely open to the uniqueness of each person's expression of reality and to have no preconceived ideas about the way in which the person's healing process would unfold.

The woman who lived on the moon was a young catatonic woman who was institutionalized. After many weeks of gaining her trust, Jung was successful in persuading her to speak. As she overcame her resistances and spoke to him, she told him that she lived on the moon. What followed was a bizarre story of what was happening on the moon and her relationship to others who lived on the moon. By listening to her story and regarding it as the absolute reality of this woman's existence, Jung was able to understand her and help her heal. After several difficult years, she was healed of her illness and lived a normal life.

The Archetypes

Looking up at the night sky, one can see figures created by patterns in the stars. Andromeda, the maiden, with her outstretched arms, Orion, the brave hunter, and a panoply of gods, goddesses, and animals cavort about the heavens. If we lived in an earlier time, we would probably sit around a fire and tell stories of these celestial inhabitants that had been passed down through generations. These stories would also be about the stars and the earth and its inhabitants; about the north wind that blows in the cold weather, and about the time that the sun disappeared. Stories were told of the hero who saved the maiden after encounters with a great beast and of gods who descended to Earth and mortals who ascended to heaven. These stories helped our ancestors understand their connection to the world around them. The stories were centered not only on basic survival needs, but also on spiritual needs and were expressions of recurrent themes or archetypes. Moreover, just as those themes had a powerful hold on our ancestors, they continue to affect us up to the present day.

We no longer sit around the campfire and tell stories, but we do sit, mesmerized for hours, in front of the flickering movie screen or television. And what we watch is, at its core, surprisingly similar to the stories our ancestors once told. The weather is still a powerful source of fascination to humans, as it was when humans depended upon knowledge of weather patterns for their survival. We no longer pay homage to the gods of thunder and lightning but are still stimulated on a deep level by the idea of a strong storm. A few winters ago, there was extensive media coverage of a predicted blizzard in the northeast United States, with forecasts of vast amounts of snow and all kinds of emergency warnings. Everyone was glued to his or her radio or television. All of the food was sold out of the grocery stores, and the story of the blizzard was on everyone's lips. As fickle nature would have it, the blizzard turned out to be a pretty small snowstorm. However, we were all left with, a very exciting media blizzard, which, I suspect, everyone thoroughly enjoyed.

As far as stories of heroes, we don't need to look any further than our latest movies, whether the hero is a super karate star or captain of a submarine or a Jedi knight, the theme is the same—the hero's journey. Hollywood stories of astronauts and starships ascending into unknown space abound, along with the ever-present aliens descending to planet Earth to either save or destroy us. These are our present day myths and stories, and if you look behind the surface of them, you will see ideas that relate to the same human concerns that are the themes of the most ancient myths and stories. Behind these themes are ideas, similar to Plato's Idea, that are preformed tendencies inherent within the human psyche.

Here we must differentiate between archetypes in their pure form and the symbolism that they stimulate. The archetypal symbol is imagery generated and regulated by the archetype, but the archetype is, in itself, invisible. It is an innate predisposition that may be an inherent component of the brain. The archetypes stimulate the individual mind to make a vast variety of images. The imagery can turn out to be the *Mona Lisa* or Monet's water lilies or some imagery straight out of "The Pit and the Pendulum" or the Marquis de Sade.

Another way to look at the archetype is to compare it to the axial system of a crystal. The axial system has the capacity to form the crystalline structure in the mother liquid, even though the axial system has no material structure of its own. It determines the basic structure of the crystal but not the ultimate size of the crystal or the exact shape. So too with the archetype. It is a predisposition toward a certain manifestation but does not specifically determine the image. As the contents of the collective unconscious, the archetypes are pre-form, pre-thought systems of readiness for action but not the actions themselves.

In becoming familiar with the imagery of myths and legends, we begin to understand some of the universal patterns contained within the archetypes and, in turn, learn at least a bit about the human psyche. However, it is not enough to rely only on information from the past; we must investigate the present meaning of the archetypes through individual dreams and visions. It is the task of each age to understand the archetypal symbols in a new way, as each age has its own challenges.

The Symbol

In order to appreciate the function of archetypal symbolism as a form of communication from the unconscious, it is important to understand what is meant by a symbol. A true symbol has no fixed meaning but, rather, points to a greater reality that can never be totally understood, because it contains wisdom that transcends the knowing mind. The symbol simply points to a greater reality and is not to be confused for the reality, as in the following Zen saying:

> *A finger is useful to point at the moon,*
> *The wise look at the moon, the ignorant at the finger.*

When a symbol becomes fixed, with a universally agreed upon meaning, it ceases to be a symbol and becomes a sign. A good example of this is the stop sign. Not only does everyone recognize it for what it is, but it is inherently limited in its agreed upon meaning. It says *stop*. A true symbol does not say *stop*, it points toward more and encourages exploration of an unknown reality.

When the meaning of a symbol is fixed by society or religion, the symbol becomes like a stone that has been lying in riverbed. The running water has removed all of the rough edges and unique shapes, and the stone becomes smooth and uniform. When we become familiar with symbols without renewing and exploring their uniqueness, we wear them out. A symbol is only alive when it is pregnant with unknown meaning. This is one of the reasons why Western society is now looking toward symbols from the East. Although thousands of years old, these symbols have a new, fresh meaning for the Western mind.

Theoretically, there is an infinite number of archetypal symbols, but some show up in the dreams and visions so often that they are more defined in Jungian psychology. The archetypes of the Self, or universal ordering factor, the shadow, and the anima in the man and the animus in the woman are the most frequently encountered. Although these archetypes are described as if they are separate and delineated, in actuality, they overlap and are never this clear. To quote Marie-Louise von Franz: "The archetypes do not swim around in the collective unconscious like pieces of bread in a soup, but rather they are the whole soup at every point and therefore always appear in specific mixtures."[3]

Not only do the archetypes overlap and interconnect with one another, but they also each have positive and negative manifestations. The understanding and acceptance of this polarity plays an important role in the process of individuation.

A few years ago, I attended a course on Japanese calligraphy taught by a master calligrapher. Our first assignment was to draw circles with brush and ink. We all struggled in our attempts to make the perfect Zen circle. After letting us sweat over this for about an hour, the instructor had us sit around and comment on our "best" circles. As each member of the class described what they liked about their circle, it became clear that we were all striving for the roundest, most spontaneous experience of circle perfection. Finally, the master calligrapher spoke to us about the exercise. The exercise was not about making the best circle, he explained, it was about wholeness. Wholeness contains not only what we like but also what we do not like. It is about the white paper as much as the black ink and our wiggly, nervous lines as well as the smooth strokes.

Like the attitude of the master calligrapher, working with the archetypes requires the presence of mind to be aware and not engulfed by the reality of the opposites. For instance, the conscious mind often idealizes the archetype of the mother although, in reality, that archetype has a more unsavory side, the dark, devouring mother in addition to the nurturing goddess. On the other hand, the shadow archetype is frequently thought of as negative, being the repository of unwanted and unaccepted qualities in ourselves. But the shadow has another side, in which hidden gifts and abilities may lie dormant until the shadow is confronted.

The awareness of the archetypes and their opposing nature allows the individual to gain more strength and stability as he or she accepts the reality of conflict and paradox within the psyche. Symbols from dreams and visions, as well as symbolic language and gestures, can point to where conflict exists. And a therapist trained in observing the symbolic realm can help the individual overcome resistance to the inevitable conflict. Acceptance and reconciliation of the reality of the opposites within the personality is an arduous process, because each time the ego is confronted with what was previously unacceptable, it struggles to maintain its former point of view. This creates inner conflict, turmoil, and even depression. When the individual finally integrates the conflict, acceptance leads to an expansion of awareness and a broadening of the personality. This ongoing expansion, combined with the development of the individual personality, is a natural process that Jung called individuation. Although Jung explored and named the process, individuation is not unique to Jungian analysis. It is a natural development that occurs in many ways, through various paths. The tendency toward individuation is an inborn potential of every human being, but only through conscious pursuance will the potential manifest. Individuation is like the Zen concept of enlightenment. Enlightenment cannot be found, because it is a sudden and spontaneous expression of what is already there, but it comes only to those who spend the time and effort looking for it.

By working with the symbolic realm, it is possible to shine some light on this process and to support others in their development. It is not easy, however, because most cultures today rely heavily, if not completely, on rational thinking as the primary form of investigating reality. Because of this bias, it is easy to dismiss the realm of symbolism and its paradoxical nature.

If we understand the nature of the archetype and its relationship to the archetypal symbol, we can then begin to understand the relationship of the archetype to human suffering and disease. The archetype is simply itself, but the relationship of the ego personality to the archetype is of utmost importance for the health of the individual. This relationship can be seen in the complexes of the individual. A complex is a bundle of emotionally charged ideas with an archetypal core. When activated, a complex upsets the usual psychic balance and functioning of an individual. The question is not if we have those complexes but how many we have and how activated they are. Our complexes are our "buttons" that are often being pushed. The idea and experience of the complex is not unique to Jungian psychology, but was originally discovered and named by Jung. What is unique about the Jungian approach to the complex is the understanding that the complex has at its core an archetype. This means that, even though the complex itself is individual, the complex's core is connected to the collective unconscious and archetypal symbolism.

The complex becomes a working model for understanding the dynamics of the whole person and the role of archetypal symbolism in the person's life. This symbolism is most easily seen in dreams and fantasies but is also present in the symbolism of bodily symptoms and sensitivities and in emotional symptoms such as fears and phobias. Symbolic manifestations of the archetype spontaneously arise during times of stress or mental breakdown, when the complex is most activated. The archetypal image often indicates that the individual is experiencing difficulty connected to a basic human problem, such as finding meaning in their life or relating to the reality of the existence of evil.

The following is an example of archetypal symbolism appearing throughout a person's life and how recognition of that symbolism helped to find a homeopathic remedy that assisted her in her healing process. M is a very intelligent and creative woman in her sixties, who has had a history of psychotic episodes. At this point in her life, she is interested in becoming as healthy as she can be. Dissatisfaction because she is misunderstood runs through her story. She has had trouble with her eyes from an early age and is now legally blind. At her first eye exam, in her forties; the doctor said she had the eyes of an eighty-five-year-old woman. Her dialogue reflects some interesting symbolism:

> *I must have seen a lot. I have looked through microscopes, video cameras, and computers. The first time I looked through the microscope, I saw the cosmos in the tissue slide I was looking at.*
>
> *I'm developing a course in mind, body, spirit interface. It's all about the order of the universe, fractals, and connections. I like to think my name stands for Minerva, who is the goddess of wisdom and crafts. She wove and spun. My first movie was about spinning and weaving.*
>
> *When I was thirty-one I slipped into a psychotic state. I was working with a very esoteric group in group therapy—they felt I was slipping away—they brought me to a psychiatrist. My pupils were dilated. They put me on Thorazine.*
>
> *I talk—but I don't feel that I am being heard. So I started studying communication. Then became interested in film.*
>
> *A year later I met my second husband, we worked together. But the relationship was difficult—the feeling of rejection was overwhelming. This marriage ended—I went to a Reichian therapist—it opened all kinds of doors—but I became psychotic again.*
>
> *Nine years later I was again given Thorazine and hospitalized.*
>
> *I am now married to my third husband. He doesn't understand me. I don't feel he is really sympathetic to who I really am. I'm cheerful on the outside but feel a deep sense of sadness inside.*
>
> *Mom was tough and tough on me. Very strict. She hit me. I was told I was too sensitive, cried too easily.*
>
> *Mom would always say how much she loved me but never let me*

express myself. After my first marriage ended–I wanted to come home but Mom wouldn't let me.

In my dreams I am always traveling–always in transit–always alone. Hard to make connections.

Once when I was hospitalized, I found this ball of black wool and I had a compulsion to weave it around the chair in my room. That black wool was so iridescent.

In her dialogue, M refers to spinning and weaving several times; she even made a film about spinning and weaving. When hospitalized during one of her psychotic episodes, she wove black yarn around a chair in her room. The yarn appeared iridescent to her. These images remind one of a spider spinning her web. She even refers to herself as Minerva. Minerva is the name of Roman goddess of wisdom, handicrafts, and arts, who is known as Athena or Pallas in ancient Greek mythology.

The myth of the goddess Minerva, as told by Ovid, includes a story about the maiden Arachne, who had such skill in the arts of weaving and embroidery that the nymphs themselves would leave their groves and fountains to gaze upon her work. Those who saw her work said that she must have been taught by Minerva herself. However, Arachne was vain about her weaving and could not bear to think of being a pupil, even to a goddess. She challenged Minerva to a contest in weaving. Minerva was very displeased by all of this and, disguised as an old woman, came down to Earth and warned Arachne not to challenge her. "Challenge your fellow mortals," she said, "but do not compete with a goddess. Ask her forgiveness for your defiance, and if she is merciful, she will forgive you."

Now, this is fair warning from the goddess about the dangers of hubris. Only those with excessive pride and ambition challenge the gods and goddesses, and pride usually leads to their downfall. A warning against hubris is warning of the dangers of identification with the archetype. Human beings are not archetypal energies; they are and must remain earthbound and ego bound to some extent. Living in the archetypal realm of the gods is dangerous to the human condition. Unconscious identification with an archetype is an overpowering experience for the ego and leads to possession by the archetype. In extreme cases, this can lead to psychosis. In M's situation, each time she moved too deeply into the archetypal realm she had a psychotic break. She, like Arachne, unknowingly commits the crime of hubris, steps over into the archetypal realm of the gods and becomes possessed by them. The story of Arachne continues:

Arachne did not heed the warning of the old woman. She stopped her spinning and turned to the old woman. "I am not afraid of the goddess, let her try her skill, if she dare." At this point Minerva drops her disguise and stands in full regalia in front of Arachne. The nymphs and bystanders bowed in reverence but Arachne maintained her foolish resolve to challenge the goddess. They proceeded to the contest.

Each of them sat at their loom and began their work. Their hands move skillfully and lightly, the excitement of the contest moving hands and shuttles easily. The colors of the wool are as the rainbows formed by sunbeams reflected from mist.

In the height of a psychotic break, M wove black wool around a chair in the hospital. She experienced it as beautifully iridescent, just like the wool in the weavings of Arachne and Minerva, the sun shining on the wool reflecting the colors of the rainbow.

Minerva wove into her web the scene of twelve heavenly powers and her contest with Neptune. She depicted herself as a war goddess with helmet and armor. In the four corners of the weaving were representations of incidents illustrating the anger of the gods when mortals presumed to challenge them. These were meant as warnings to Arachne to give up the contest before it was too late.

Arachne covered her web with designs chosen to show the failings and errors of the gods. It was beautifully depicted but irreverent and arrogant. Minerva could not help but admire the work but felt indignant at the insult. She struck Arachne's weaving with her shuttle, tearing it into pieces. She then touched Arachne's forehead with the shuttle, making her feel guilt and shame. Arachne could not endure it, went and hanged herself.

Minerva pitied her as she saw her suspended by her rope. She brought her to life by sprinkling her with Aconite and turning her into a spider. Arachne continues to live, spinning her thread and, often hanging suspended, as she was when Minerva touched her and transformed her into a spider.[4]

According to Massimo Mangialavori, the web-weaving spider, *Aranea diadema,* is a remedy for people who need to define their own identity. He explains that the feeling of not having been understood and appreciated for what and who they are is more predominant in people who need this remedy. Unfortunately, these people often search for support from their families, and their families are often unable to understand or help. Even worse, people who need this remedy have the tendency to reproduce this lack of understanding in their own relationships, falling in love with people that show a very similar behavior to that of their families. These people find themselves in a position in which they fight for identity in front of a family and society that never even recognized them as an individual person.[5]

Because of her many associations to weaving and to the archetype of the spider, along with her feelings of being misunderstood, M was given *Aranea diadema.*

After a few months on the remedy, her confidence and feeling of dissatisfaction at being misunderstood were greatly improved. She has not had any psychotic breaks and is moving forward with her work over the last two years. She now has better relationships and no longer feels that people have to understand her completely. The result of her homeopathic treatment is best explained in her own words:

> *Since I took the remedy, I've been walking on the bottom of my own pond. My relationship with my husband is more peaceful—I know that he doesn't have to understand everything.*
>
> *Sometimes my thoughts had become too big for this little body. I'm learning not to get so abstract. My breakdowns were always very creative. They were brought about by a huge amount of rage—rage caused by the feeling that trust was betrayed. I don't have that component anymore now. I can feel the joy of being in touch with very deep spaces in myself. Previously, I tried to do things that I couldn't accomplish.*

Relationship to the Archetype

Perception of what needs to be healed in an individual is of paramount importance in any healing relationship. We cannot proceed in any healing modality without some idea of the goal of the therapy. The truth of the matter, however, is that it takes a lot of time and work on the part of the therapist and the patient to reach the core of what needs to be healed. In M's situation, we have some strong clues in her association to Minerva, the goddess of spinning and weaving, and to the specific story of the contest between Minerva and Arachne. Finally, we have the symbolism of the spider that was the homeopathic remedy that helped her.

The myth of Minerva is that she sprang fully armored from the head of Zeus. This is similar to creative work that springs forth from the collective unconscious fully formed. It is a kind of higher logic. This type of creativity is a gift and, at the same time, a great difficulty for the individual upon whom the gift has been bestowed. Working with the gifted individual requires an understanding of his or her particular dilemma. M is an extremely creative person who, like many creative people, felt that people did not appreciate and understand what she was trying to communicate. The dilemma in these cases is that often what they have to say is new and unfamiliar to those around them It takes a lot of ego strength to feel comfortable with the reality that many, if not the entire society, will reject your ideas. The challenge is to continue creative exploration in spite of the rejection.

The myth of Minerva that is more specifically related to M though, is the story of Minerva and Arachne, especially the weaving and the spider. The spider is an ancient archetypal symbol appearing in the creation myths of many cultures. In Navajo creation myth, Grandmother Spider Woman spins all life from the shimmering threads in her belly. Spinning and weaving is traditionally a feminine art, and many goddesses are shown spinning and weaving the universe. Plato had a dream of great goddess Ananke, "Necessity," spinning the universe; the sun, moon, and planets were her spindle's whorls; sirens sang through the webs of time and fate that she wove; and souls endlessly moved through the strands on their way to and from death and rebirth.

The ancient Vedic philosophy of India suggests that a spider wove the veil of illusion that conceals the supreme reality. In West Africa, Anansi, the spider, prepared the material from which the first humans were made and created the sun, the moon, and the stars. The spiderweb is associated with the idea of the web of life, which represents the interconnectedness and interdependence of all things. M has always had that kind of vision. Her challenge has been to integrate it into her individual, ego-bound self in such a way that she can continue to function in this world.

The art of perceiving the individual's connection to an archetype requires that the therapist understands the unique way that the personal material of the complex relates to the archetypal core. The therapist must also understand the uniqueness of the time in which the individual is living. Different eras have different challenges, and archetypal symbolism becomes enriched with changes in human development. Understanding the relationship between the personal and the archetypal within the era it is experienced gives an appreciation of new ideas and developments emerging from each individual life. It also helps to put the complexity of disease and healing into a different perspective.

In M's case, the spider and its web relates to the archetype of wholeness, a central unifying archetype that Jung called the Self. More specifically, we are dealing with the archetype of the Self in a feminine form, as the creative goddess spinning the web of the universe. At times, M's mind would go so far into the reality of this archetype that she could not contain it. It was at those times that she would experience a psychotic break. In a situation like this, the most important help that can be given is to strengthen the individual ego self (as opposed to the archetypal Self) so that it can withstand this level of reality. It is also important to break the inappropriate enthrallment with the archetypal realm.

Fascination with the archetypal realm is very dangerous. In the myth, Arachne is warned by Minerva not to challenge the gods. Another way of saying this is not to play with the gods. Humans must remain in the human sphere. If we stray too far into the world of the gods, there is a great danger of losing one's human self. In unconscious identification with an archetype, one is in danger of becoming possessed by the archetype and losing one's autonomy. One may also be either overinflated or demolished by an energy that is impossible for an individual to contain.

The goal is to improve the awareness of the ego self in relationship to the archetype. In doing so, it is possible to be in relationship to the archetype and understand that the realm of the gods belongs to the gods. We can then learn to operate with our feet on the ground and one eye on the heavens. The gods are willing to assist us as long as we understand our place.

M was at first too deeply identified with the archetypal realm. Her challenge was to ground herself more deeply in the here and now. For others, who are more earthbound, connection with the timeless realm of the collective unconscious can create a new perspective on life. This connection sometimes comes in unexpected ways and can be delivered by unusual messengers.

A while back, some friends were sitting around the fireplace in my living room when Jim, who is an artist and environmentalist, told us an interesting story. About ten years ago, he was camping in a remote area and came upon a moss-covered rock. The moss had formed in such a way that it looked like a frog sitting in the middle of a fire. Jim was so impressed with this that he made a drawing of it, but he didn't think much more about it until our discussion.

I was aware enough of the parallel between Jim's frog picture and the alchemical drawings of salamanders surrounded by fire to know that this image was symbolic of a transformational process. Jim and I talked about it for a while. He related it to his environmental concerns, thinking that, perhaps it was a sign about frogs being wiped out by environmental pollutants. I asked him to look further into his own relationship to the frog in the fire. Was this a message from the collective unconscious stimulating a much-needed transformation? We didn't come to any answer, just more questions.

In working with archetypes and the symbolic realm, coming up with more questions is a good thing. The worst thing we can do is to pin things down too quickly. Jim was interested enough in the symbol to continue mulling it over, and he came to the decision that what he wanted to draw the frog again and have it tattooed onto his body.

Tattooing is a way that many societies have used meaningful symbols for thousands of years. The symbol becomes a permanent and integral part of the body, thus linking the body to the archetypal realm through the sacred symbol or totem.

I didn't hear from Jim for a while, but he did get his tattoo. A few months later he very excitedly told me the following story. He went to an old friend of his who is a tattoo artist. The tattoo artist loved his drawing and, being familiar with Jim's other artwork, suggested that his style would lend itself very well to tattoo. The result of all this was that Jim gave up a job working in an office and started working as a tattoo artist. He is spending a lot more of his time on his artwork now, drawing on human easels as well as paper and canvas.

Jim opened himself to the symbol of the frog in the fire, a symbol of the heat of the transformation process that is necessary for alchemical change. In doing this, he also opened himself up to his own creativity and the expression of his art. Finding the rock with the image of a frog was an example of synchronicity, that mysterious connection between the personal psyche and the material world. It served as a messenger that, when given its due, served as a vehicle for change.

Messages from the symbolic realm are all around us. They appear in nature, in dreams and visions, and in bodily symptoms. Too often, they are judged with the rational mind and the precious gift is ignored. We tend to consider ourselves beyond what our inner nature gives freely and believe that answers come only from some man-made, institutionalized source outside of ourselves. The result of ignoring messages from the deeper realms of the psyche, the basis of the interconnectedness between humanity and nature, is already taking its toll on the health of our bodies and the state of this planet. It is time to move into the next stage of our development and elegantly integrate rational, scientific advances with the wisdom of the ages that can be found in the symbolic realm of the archetypes.

CHAPTER FIVE

The Shadow
The Guard at the Door

Man stands in his own shadow and wonders why it is dark.

ZEN SAYING

Just as all objects under a light have a shadow, the human mind has a light or conscious side and a dark unconscious side. Jung named this dark side of the mind the shadow and called it "that hidden, repressed, for the most part inferior and guilt-laden personality whose ultimate ramifications reach back into the realm of our animal ancestors and so comprise the whole historical aspect of the unconscious."[1]

As the accumulation of everything that an individual refuses to acknowledge or is unable to see in himself, the shadow contains negative qualities that cannot be faced, such as faults and bad habits, and positive qualities that are unable to be acknowledged. The shadow may also contain personal gifts and abilities that have been unaccepted by parents and society during the childhood socialization process. If, for instance, a man is taught that being yielding and sensitive is not acceptable, he may suppress those qualities, even though those qualities may be exactly what he needs to express his creativity.

Social pressure may also cause a person to suppress certain qualities. A society that abhors any type of aggressive behavior will cause many individuals to put anger and aggression in the shadow. Qualities and emotions that lie in the shadow are not directly accessible to the individual or to society but eventually seep out in uncontrollable and often destructive ways. A method of accessing these energies is to investigate the contents of the shadow, thus integrating them into the conscious mind.

While investigating shadow material can be a humbling and sometimes depressing experience, those who are able to tolerate the work reap the rewards of increased clarity and vitality. Attributes that remain in the shadow contain a great deal of personal energy that cannot be used for the benefit of the individual and may even be the source of disease. Integrating previously unconscious shadow material into the conscious mind allows the mind and body to access that energy.

The Illusory Life—Projection of the Shadow

Parts of the shadow that are not brought into conscious awareness are projected out into the world. Although the other contents of the unconscious may be transferred, it is the projection of the shadow that is of particular concern. When the shadow is projected, its unaccepted contents are blamed on others. In this unconscious state, what is denied in the inner state is seen in objects of hatred and aversion in the outside world. Because the unrealized shadow is not known to the conscious mind, the source of this transmittal is not the individual ego but the unconscious. Thus, the unconscious shadow material casts itself out onto the environment, creating an illusory world that the ego is fooled into seeing as reality. The effect of unexamined projection is, according to Jung, "to isolate the subject from his environment, since instead of a real relationship there is now only an illusory one."[2]

In other words, projections create a waking dream from which the individual is unable to emerge without significant effort. Projection of the shadow is similar to the phenomenon that in the East is called Maya, the veil of illusion. The object of many Eastern spiritual practices is to break through this veil into the reality of life. An example of this can be seen in the following discussion between a practitioner of meditation and his teacher. The practitioner, who was having a lot of trouble with his life, described many of the terrible things that were happening to him. The teacher replied, "This is your movie. Why did you decide to make it a horror film?" This reply seems at first to lack compassion, but it may have been just what the student needed to begin to question the illusion that was being created by his unconscious mind.

Only a very few will be able to accomplish the withdrawal of projection that is the goal of such spiritual practice, but awareness of the projection of the personal shadow is a goal that can be reached by many. The personal shadow is the repository of an individual's unwanted and unconscious material, the exploration of which is most often the first step in healing. When the personal shadow is integrated, there is less likelihood of projecting its contents onto the environment and the surroundings appear to change in surprising ways. How many times have we heard someone who has gone through a profound healing say that they have noticed an improvement in their friends or spouse? Many people exclaim that, suddenly, after years of unpleasantness, their partner is being friendlier and more loving, or that they have gotten a new job, or that things have miraculously changed in their old job. Never mind that these things had been going on in the same way for years; it is now suddenly different. Has the world now conspired to help these people, where in the past it was working against them? No. What has been altered is within themselves, and that change is projected out onto their environment.

Jung's concept of projection is very similar to the homeopathic view of the development of symptoms. Homeopathic philosophy states that symptoms are generated by the vital force, the symptoms flowing outward from a previously deranged inner state. In his *Lectures on Homeopathic Philosophy*, James Tyler Kent, the great American homeopath who lived and practiced into the early twentieth century, describes this process:

> The internal state of man is prior to that which surrounds him, therefore, environment is not the cause; it is only, as it were, a sounding board; it only reacts upon and reflects the internal. . . . Diseases correspond to man's affections, and the diseases that are upon the human race today are but the outward expression of man's interiors, and it is true if the diseases are such they represent the internal forces of man. Man hates his neighbour, he is willing to violate every commandment; such is the state of man today. This state is represented in man's diseases. All diseases upon the earth, acute and chronic, are representations of man's internals. Otherwise he could not be susceptible, or could not develop that which is within him. The image of his own interior self comes out in disease.[3]

Here, Kent tells us that the internal state is prior to and contributes to the development of physical disease. He writes that an individual's interior state is seen in the imagery of the disease and in the person's attitude toward the outside world. Although Kent focuses more on the development of physical disease than does Jung, they are both saying that the inner state creates the outer state. The understanding of the role of the inner state creating bodily disease is more developed in homeopathy, through

Hahnemann's miasmatic theory, and the mechanism of the inner state or psyche is more deeply understood in Jungian psychology. The homeopathic theory of miasms states that in order for someone to fall ill to a particular disease, there must be an underlying state of illness that predisposes them toward disease. According to Hahnemann, miasms are characteristic of the underlying disease that afflicts most of humanity, being passed on from generation to generation unless cured by a method of treatment, like homeopathy, that addresses this root cause of disease. Because miasmatic theory deals with an underlying and collective condition of humanity, it has much in common with Jung's concept of the collective unconscious.

The effect of the unconscious on the individual and the individual's environment can be compared to the primary importance of the immune system in the maintenance of health, rather than disease being a function of the onslaught of external pathogens and influences only. In both cases, the individual's internal state can be overridden by external factors, but it is essential to understand that the internal state plays an important role in creating the status quo of the individual.

The relationship between the internal state and disease is not a simple relationship between the conscious mind, the body, and the environment. It has become fashionable in some circles to speak about such things in an overly simplistic way, so that the individual appears to be responsible for his or her own disease. If this were so, all a person would have to do is think differently in order to cure his or her disease. To accuse an individual of creating disease is misguided and insulting. What is being discussed here is an interior state that exists previous to thought and is not under the control of the conscious mind.

Projection of preconscious, previously encoded material is what serves as reality, to a greater or lesser extent, for everyone. Projection also colors the symptoms of physical and mental disease. While it is impossible to escape this phenomenon, the homeopath must recognize that projection exists if he or she is to objectively evaluate the situation of an individual, perceive what needs to be healed, and find the appropriate remedy.

Acquaintance with the shadow is the first step in an appreciation of this phenomenon, for the shadow stands at the door to greater knowledge, forbidding entry to those who will not confront this archetype. Because unexplored shadow material masks the inner landscape, as well as the external state, it is impossible to objectively evaluate the state of another person until the personal shadow is acknowledged and at least partially integrated.

The Collective Shadow

On first encountering the shadow there is no differentiation between what is personal and what belongs to the collective unconscious, but as one becomes more conscious of shadow material it becomes clear that aspects of it do not belong to the individual alone. One begins to differentiate and understand the larger picture; the collective shadow.

Every community, country, and culture has its collective shadow that it projects out onto others. In biblical times, communities would often perform rituals in which a goat representing all that was evil and negative in the community, i.e., the shadow of the community, was sent out into the desert to die. This is the derivation of the word *scapegoat.* We can also say that a scapegoat is a person, country, or culture that serves as the object of the projected collective shadow.

Guiseppe Tornatore portrays this phenomenon in the Italian film *Malena.* The film takes place in a small Sicilian town during World War II, where a beautiful young woman, Malena, becomes the object of desire of most of the town's male population. The combined focus of sexual energy leads to jealous and malicious gossip about Malena that builds up until she is beaten by the women of the village and forced to leave. It is a story of sexual suppression and what happens to that unexpressed energy accumulated within the collective shadow. The collective shadow must have some object on which to express itself. In this case the shadow is projected onto a young woman and affects her life in a profound way.

Countries also have a collective shadow and a need to project that shadow. People are usually unaware of the shadow of their own country, except through another country that is perceived as an enemy. When negative energy builds up to the point at which it can no longer be contained, it is released through explosions of violence or even war. Ancient civilizations often used rituals such as the scapegoat ritual in biblical times or other types of sacrifice to assuage this buildup in the collective unconscious. Contemporary society has felt the need to cleanse itself of such "barbaric" rituals, but the need to deal with the collective shadow remains.

As we move into the twenty-first century, a development is taking place that requires a change in the way that humanity has been dealing with the collective shadow. Through increased communication and air travel, we have become more of a global community, and it is much more dangerous to project our collective shadow onto another country. The threat of nuclear war has put us all in the same soup. We are now a global community, whether we like it or not. What do we do with our shadow energy as it becomes more and more life-threatening to project it? The time has come for a development in consciousness that leads to a different way of dealing with shadow energy.

One aspect of this development is for each of us to take responsibility for our own shadow in order to alleviate the buildup of negativity within the collective shadow. If this is to be done, it leads to some very special challenges for therapists and health practitioners. It requires that those in the healing arts process their own shadow material and understand the role of the shadow in health and disease.

Recently, there has been an increase in health problems that cannot be successfully treated, such as autoimmune diseases, cancer, and AIDS. Many types of medications, such as antibiotics, that address disease organisms are no longer effective against many acute diseases. Obesity and infertility are continuing to increase. These trends may indicate the need to look in another direction to evaluate the causes of these conditions.

An understanding of the shadow of the patient, the therapist, and medicine in general will be one way to give insight into these problems. Many questions are still unanswered in this area and must be dealt with, ultimately, on an individual level. Too little is known about the role of the shadow in disease, but it is certain that we cannot begin to understand this problem until the shadow, both collective and personal, is brought further into the light of consciousness.

Prescribing on the Shadow and Case Analysis

Understanding the client and perceiving what needs to be healed is one of the most important parts of successful homeopathic treatment. It requires that the homeopath be able to gather enough accurate information from the initial interview on which to base the prescription. The initial interview, or case taking, is an art as well as a science. Its efficacy is improved if the homeopath is familiar with the idea of the shadow in addition to knowledge of standard homeopathic case taking. Very often, the true nature of an individual is hidden in deep shadow material, under the cover of a mask or persona. If we prescribe based on the "face value" of this mask, we will be far away from prescribing a remedy that will help the individual. A sweet, yielding persona can mask an indifferent and cruel nature, and a tough exterior may be covering an insecure and timid disposition.

A person disguising deep shadow material under the mask of the persona will often have an immobile or masklike face. They may also appear to be too nice or be too good to be true, or the practitioner may feel that the person is not telling the whole story. This should set off a red light to the homeopath, especially when the "too nice" individual has a history of a terrible childhood or if others have mistreated them. In these cases, the homeopath must look deeper, into other areas where the true essence of the individual may be seen.

The shadow can often be seen in dreams, which tend to compensate for the conscious state. It may appear as a person of the same sex as the dreamer and have a dark, black, or primitive quality. The shadow can also appear in the form of a person the dreamer particularly dislikes. In a person who is cruel and even criminal, the shadow may appear in dreams that are light and sweet. In contrast, a very holy and saintlike person may have lascivious or violent dreams that indicate their opposite side.

Favored activities, such as reading material and movies, may reveal the shadow of an individual, especially if these activities stand in contrast to the more conscious state. The mild-mannered pacifist who loves to go to violent movies is expressing his or her shadow through this activity. A creative artist who expresses herself through gory paintings or writings, even though she wouldn't consider such activities in her everyday life, is expressing something important about her unconscious, suppressed side. One can often tell a lot about a person by looking at their artwork. Children's art is particularly graphic in showing the shadow, and looking at their drawings is an effective tool in gathering symptoms.

Once the homeopath becomes accustomed to seeing the shadow of individuals through their facial expression, dreams, and activities, he or she can begin to see even more subtle manifestations of the shadow. Often, the shadow will be so deeply hidden that it emerges only in the symptoms of disease and in subtle symptoms that can only be seen when viewed in relation to the disease or to the dream state.

For example, Jeffrey, who appears to be very haughty and closed, is interviewed for homeopathic treatment. The homeopath finds that Jeffrey is very sympathetic and concerned with injustice. These qualities, along with his arthritic tendency and indifference to sweets, remind the homeopath of the remedy *Causticum.* But Jeffrey's present problem is kidney stones, with a history of prolapse of the kidney. Since his general state seems to be so similar to *Causticum,* do we give it and hope it works for the kidney stones? But *Causticum* is also not indicated for the prolapse.

A repertorization (cataloging and research) of his symptoms shows several main remedies, including *Phosphorus, Belladonna,* and *Colocynthus.* The clinical experience of many homeopaths indicates that *Colocynthus* is a complementary remedy to *Causticum,* so *Colocynthus* is a possibility. *Phosphorus* covers many of his symptoms, but also doesn't cover the prolapse. Which remedy to use is still unclear.

The homeopath notes that Jeffrey had his first encounter with kidney stone colic many years before, after losing his job. In going back and more carefully questioning him about that time, the homeopath finds that Jeffrey was angry at losing a job that he liked. Although he says nothing about resentment at this time, the most closely indicated remedy is one for ailments from anger, *Colocynthus.*

What was hidden in the shadow becomes clearer as the correct remedy emerges and the homeopath can now see that the theme of anger runs throughout the case. But the anger is expressed in such a subtle way that it could not be seen at first. Looking back on the case, the homeopath now remembers that Jeffrey complained about the condition of the waiting room, refused to answer certain questions pertaining to his anger, and that there was a subtle but pervasive feeling of irritation during the interview. This is typical of an emotion that is hidden in the shadow. It is a submerged emotion that leaks out and may be felt by the homeopath, even though the patient does not directly express it.

Another way for the homeopath to get a peek at what is going on in the shadow is through the patient's projection of the individual's shadow onto others. Qualities that are disliked or hated in others are often the qualities of an individual's own shadow. If, during the interview, a patient mentions that she hates her father, the homeopath can ask what qualities the father has that are so disliked. Finding out about the personality of the father can lead to some interesting symptoms that are shared by both the patient and the father. In the patient, they are hidden in the shadow. If one of the remedies indicated by the physical and general symptoms is known for the hated symptoms of the father, it may be the correct remedy for the patient.

For example, the case of Martha (not an actual case, but a composite of cases) demonstrates the use of the shadow in homeopathic practice. Martha's physical symptoms indicate the need for *Nitric acid. Nitric acid* is well known for its use in people who have negative personality traits such as hatred, holding grudges, and blaming everyone. However, Martha is very sweet and never blames anyone for anything. As a matter of fact, she

has a very strongly held philosophy of always maintaining a positive outlook on life. This may indicate that *Nitric acid* is the wrong remedy for the
patient.

When the homeopath questions Martha about who in her life is a very
difficult person, she mentions her aunt Grady. When asked why this aunt is
a problem for her, she replies that she cannot bear to be around her, because the aunt is always blaming everyone for her problems, is extremely
negative, and never forgives anyone for even the slightest offense. Aunt
Grady appears, at least to Martha, to have the negative qualities indicating
the use of *Nitric acid.*

It may be that the aunt's symptoms are a projection of Martha's shadow.
Why else would she consider her to be the most difficult person in her life?
When coupled with Martha's "too good to be true" commitment to a
positive outlook, the disliked aunt's qualities point to a shadow that contains the qualities indicating the use of *Nitric acid.*

Martha may also have repeated dreams of evil people who hate her or of
being brought to trial as a criminal. These dreams may also indicate the
shadow part of her personality that, along with her physical symptoms,
resonates with *Nitric acid.*

The homeopath may find it useful to apply the concept of the shadow to
understanding remedies. Looking again at *Nitric acid,* it may come as a surprise to see that the provings of this remedy contain, along with the typical
negative symptoms, the following more positive symptoms: cheerfulness, gaiety,
general happiness, desire for company, ecstasy, impressionable, susceptible, mirth,
hilarity, liveliness, sympathetic, and compassionate.

Because knowledge of what can be cured by a homeopathic remedy is
gleaned from the experiences of human beings in provings, poisonings, and
clinical experience, the remedies will contain some opposing symptoms.
These opposing symptoms are the symptoms of the shadow. Every remedy
that is understood through the human mind and body must, necessarily, be
two-sided. Referring back to the provings will reveal this. A remedy only
appears to be one-sided because one side is better known than the other.

When homeopaths first learn materia medica, they are usually taught
that the remedy *Anacardium* is for hardened, cruel people who are capable
of malicious deeds and violent behavior (along with their lack of confidence). But how many of these types of people would be interested in
homeopathic treatment? And, yet, *Anacardium* is an important and widely
used remedy. Is it that it has been prescribed mainly on its physical indications of sensation of a plug, amelioration from eating, and skin eruptions?

If so, what is the relationship between the mental symptoms in the materia medica and the practical use of the remedy?

In fact, many of the people who need *Anacardium* have an inability to express anger. However, they may have extremely violent dreams and fantasies. On the other hand, their anger may be deeply submerged, oozing out from time to time in the sinister way that the shadow expresses itself. In those who need this remedy, there is a great division between the conscious state and the unconscious shadow. The shadow is seen in the delusions of those who need *Anacardium*. That includes the delusion that mind and body are separated, and a devil whispers in the individual's ear.

Becoming familiar with the concept and the reality of the shadow will help homeopaths to more fully understand the often paradoxical proving symptoms in the homeopathic materia medica. This knowledge will also help in understanding what needs to be healed in the patient without being so easily fooled by a persona that hides the underlying personal traits so important in locating the correct remedy.

Ultimately, the homeopath should examine his or her own shadow, to more clearly differentiate the practitioner's own projections from the actual situation of the patient. If homeopaths are not aware of their shadows, they may project them out onto their clients. This may prevent the homeopaths from clearly seeing what needs to be cured, because each person they come in contact with will be colored by the practitioners' own shadow issues. For example, if a homeopath, while overtly friendly, has a great deal of unconscious animosity toward human beings, this animosity will be projected outward onto his or her clients, and they will feel nervous and anxious in the homeopath's presence. Because they feel uncomfortable, they will not be able to divulge their inner feelings and sensations. The homeopath, in turn, will end up thinking that most of the clients are very nervous and anxious and will overprescribe remedies that are appropriate for anxious people.

Even worse, unconscious shadow material from the homeopath may be "dumped" onto the client, leaving the client feeling angry, depressed, or in some other negative state. If the homeopath has, for instance, a great deal of unconscious anxiety about health (a common quality in health-care practitioners—that is why they get into a profession where they can think about it all the time), this feeling may be instilled into the client. Some practitioners feel so anxious about health that their clients cannot get well until they leave them and go to someone who can cleanse them of the infection.

One way that homeopaths can get a glimpse of their shadow is to look at what remedies they prescribe much more frequently than other remedies.

Whether these are accurate prescriptions or not, they may give a clue to the homeopath's shadow. This does not mean that the homeopath necessarily needs the remedy but rather that the homeopath continually perceives certain qualities in others that are indicative of his or her shadow.

Keeping a dream journal and working with a dream partner is helpful, for dreams often show the shadow. More detailed information on working with one's own dreams is included in chapter 7 of this book. For those homeopaths who have the opportunity, working with a psychologist or analyst who will help them see their shadow material is one of the best ways to keep this unconscious material from contaminating the therapeutic relationship.

The first step in working with the shadow is to realize that it exists—that each person has a shadow and it can be projected out onto others. To recognize that this dynamic is a part of one's own interaction with clients already brings light onto the problem. However the homeopath then chooses to work with the shadow, it is no easy feat, for, as Jung writes, the shadow is "a moral problem that challenges the whole ego-personality, for no one can become conscious of the shadow without considerable effort."[4]

CHAPTER SIX

Anima/Animus

Male and Female

Male and female represent the two sides of the great radical dualism. But in fact they are perpetually passing into one another. Fluid hardens to solid, solid rushes to fluid. There is no wholly masculine man, no purely feminine woman.

MARGARET FULLER, *Woman in the Nineteenth Century,* 1845

Homeopaths who understand the implications of the shadow have the potential to assist people who would not ordinarily be able to accomplish the feat of confronting their shadow. They can support the individual through the process of integrating the shadow and know when it is necessary to refer a client to a therapist who can provide more assistance. The appropriate homeopathic remedy is a powerful tool for stimulating the healing process and unlocking blockages to awareness of the shadow. In these cases, some people will get to the laudable point of accessing another archetypal configuration within the psyche—the archetype of the anima or animus. Jung wrote, "If the encounter with the shadow is the 'apprentice-piece' in the individual's development, then that with the anima is the 'master-piece.' The relation with the anima is again a test of courage, an ordeal by fire for the spiritual and moral forces of man."[1]

The ordeal by fire to which Jung refers is the pain that is experienced when the individual is exposed to various aspects of the psyche, including the shadow and the animus and, ultimately, to the Self. When first exposed to the archetypes of the psyche, the ego identifies with and is contaminated by them. This leads to a period of depression or a "dark night of the soul," when the person must reevaluate who they are. This depression is a normal period of development and must not be confused with pathological depression. It is always a blow to the ego to be confronted with the shadow, and the encounter with the anima or animus may be equally if not more difficult, because it brings up more fundamental and subtle issues.

Whenever healing is profound enough to create a transformation there is usually a period of depression. Illustrations from alchemical archives graphically show this depression as a king sitting in a hole with a raven on his head or being beaten to death or through images of death represented by skeletons. This stage was known in alchemy as the nigredo, or referred to as *mortificatio* or *putrefactio* and represents the procedure a substance underwent in the alchemical laboratory, as well as the psychological state of the alchemist as he went through his personal transformation. It is necessary to go through this darkness, according to the alchemists, because without darkness the light could not be born. Without the substance being blackened or putrefied it would not be purified and develop the white or albedo stage. In his *Hermetic and Alchemical Writings*, Paracelsus describes the putrefactio:

> *Putrefaction is of so great efficacy that it blots out the old nature and transmutes everything into another new nature, and bears another new fruit. All living things die in it, all dead things decay, and then all these dead things regain life. Putrefaction takes away the acridity from all corrosive spirits of salt, renders them soft and sweet.*[2]

According to Paracelsus, during the putrefactio, old ideas, the old nature, is transmuted into something new. What was once acrid becomes sweet. In the light of this discussion, this transformation is the result of having encountered an archetype such as the anima or animus, allowing it to contaminate the ego and then integrating it into the conscious state. In order to facilitate this integration, it is helpful for the homeopath to be able to recognize the putrefactio and understand the shadow, the anima, and the animus.

The anima and animus, or syzygy, as they were referred to by Jung, constitute an archetype of duality because it is the inner and opposite sex of the individual. The anima is the inner feminine side of a man, and the animus the inner masculine side of a woman. According to Jung, the anima could be compared to a man's soul. The animus functions as something like the unconscious mind in a woman, but at times, Jung referred to the animus as the soul of a woman.

The syzygy is a complex, meaning that it is a conglomeration of feeling-toned ideas centered on an archetype. It can project itself out onto the environment just as the shadow projects itself. Actually, Jung felt that the anima or animus is the projection-making function of the psyche. When the projection of anima overrides the conscious will of the individual, the force of the complex dominates him. In these cases, the individual is as if possessed by the anima or animus. This is known in Jungian psychology as anima or animus possession and is one of the primary causes of difficulty in relationships.

The anima and animus can also be a positive force, functioning as a bridge between the conscious and unconscious parts of the personality. They also act like inner personalities, compensating for the personality that is experienced consciously by the individual and seen by the outside world.

Being a male, Jung wrote much more about the anima, because he understood it from his personal experience. In addition, although he must have frequently encountered the animus in clinical practice, many of his views of its function were strongly colored by the patriarchal prejudices of his time. Since the author, being a woman, suffers from a similar predicament of needing to rely on personal experience, the following is weighted rather heavily toward the animus.

The animus is the repository of all of a woman's ancestral experiences of the masculine and has not only an individual but also a collective aspect. The greater access a woman has to the collective unconscious, the more her animus will be imbued with characteristics belonging to the history of the masculine spirit. Since this history is extremely complex and convoluted, and because the role of the animus in the feminine psyche is not well understood, a woman undertaking the exploration of her masculine side is endeavoring groundbreaking work. Each woman will have a unique experience of her animus and will more than likely confront many of the prejudices about what it means to be a woman.

There are, however, some guidelines from Jung about the animus that may be very helpful to the homeopath who is following the healing process, especially Jung's idea of the four phases of the animus that follow the psychological development of this archetype. These phases may often be seen in dreams and fantasies and in the woman's relationship to the men in her life as she moves into greater wholeness under homeopathic treatment. The animus is a collective figure, and it is possible for a woman to have strong associations to the animus at more than one level of development, and any of these aspects can be projected out onto a man or in some cases onto another woman.

In the first and most primitive stage, the animus appears as an embodiment of physical power. He may appear as a superhero or muscle man or, if the woman has a particularly ugly association with men, as a brutal criminal type. These animus figures may be seen in her dreams and fantasies, or be reflected in the types of men that she is drawn to. The presence of this type of animus explains why many women are attracted to men with whom they appear to have nothing in common. A very sophisticated woman may date a beer drinking construction worker who prefers to watch wrestling on television, while she is drawn to the opera. Her friends can't imagine what she sees in him, but, because he is a reflection of her animus, he may resonate perfectly with her.

Despite the opinion of friends and society, as long as a woman has a positive relationship with her animus, relationships with men who resonate with this stage of the animus are not a problem. They only become so if the animus is especially negative. In addition, any level of the animus can be projected onto a man, contaminating the woman's view of him and leading to unrealized expectations. She may wish for him to be her knight in shining armor while he, like most people, simply wants to get on with his life. On the other hand, she may project the negative traits of her animus onto him, accusing him of undeserved actions and attitudes.

Unfortunately, because the history of the relationship between men and women is both personally and collectively riddled with abuse and patriarchal domination of the feminine, the animus is contaminated with this energy, and most women must struggle to free themselves from its negative influence. Once she is able to free herself of some of this negative energy, a woman begins to reap the rewards of greater freedom and success in life.

At the next stage of development, the animus provides the woman with greater independence and gives her the capacity for planned action and success in the world. When the animus begins to develop into this stage, a woman's dreams and fantasies may change, so the animus appears as a more helpful figure. Her focus in life may change, and she may become more creative and interested in her own goals. Her relationship to men may also undergo a change. A different type of man may appeal to her, or her relationship with her present partner may alter dramatically. If a woman has worked through the healing process to make her animus more conscious, she will be less likely to project the negative animus onto the men in her life.

The stage that follows is the development of wisdom, and here the animus is seen in dreams and fantasies as the scholar, professor, or clergyman. The ideal man of a woman whose animus is on this level is a man who appears to have developed some wisdom. She may, at this phase, seek out a man who can serve as a mentor or may rely wholly on her internal wisdom, especially if the animus has developed to this level through an arduous healing process.

A woman whose animus has always functioned on this level is significantly different from one who has achieved this level through the healing process. One difference is that someone who has moved through the first stages will be much more aware of the animus and is familiar with the other stages. This woman will have suffered and acknowledged that much of her suffering was a projection of her own animus. Because of this, she exudes a different type of wisdom, more experienced and grounded than other women with this stage of animus development. Being more conscious of her animus, she will also be less likely to project it onto a man.

The fourth stage of the animus is as the incarnation of spiritual experience and may appear in dreams and fantasies as a messenger of the gods. This messenger may be in the form the god Hermes, of a man, or perhaps a bird, representing the movement earthward from the sky. When the animus is on this level, a woman is attracted to men who are involved in spiritual work, such as gurus, priests, and others claiming spiritual attainment. If the animus remains unconscious, the danger is that she will mistake the man on whom she projects her animus for her own ability for spiritual realization.

The integration of the animus at this level, or perhaps on other levels also, allows for changes within the individual woman that are, at the present day, largely unrealized. Until fairly recently, the roles of women were stringently held in place, so no one knows where the development of the woman in relation to her animus may lead. Since, traditionally, most religions have projected spiritual enlightenment onto a male figure, it may be that the integration of the spiritual animus may lead to a change in the way that women experience their spiritual life. If a woman no longer has the need to project her animus onto a man, she may no longer need to perceive the center of her spiritual life as a projection onto a male deity or, for that matter, a female deity.

The anima in a man is both the personal and archetypal image of woman, a composite of every woman he has known since infancy. The anima is every mother, seductress, goddess, and witch that has been represented in human consciousness throughout time. In a man's dreams and fantasies, the anima may appear as any image of woman, from lover to spiritual guide. As with the animus in the woman, the man projects his anima onto the women around him, creating a fantasy relationship that can rarely, if ever, be fulfilled by the actual woman.

While any man's anima can lead him astray and into chaos, his work with her will gradually lead him to the point at which he can appreciate her wisdom. As with the animus, Jung described four stages of the anima. The ideal situation is for the anima of a man to develop naturally as he progresses from infancy to old age. In reality, this rarely happens, and the anima ends up compensating for the conscious state of the individual. No matter what the man's stage of development, however, if the anima remains uncon- scious, everything she stands for is projected and the man searches for that development in the outside world. The most frequent object of this projec- tion is a woman and, if the man is in a relationship, his partner. Because no woman can fulfill the fantasy associated with the anima, this projection ends with predictably disastrous results.

In naming the four stages of the anima, Jung drew on previous associa- tions to stages of eroticism in myth and literature: Eve, Helen of Troy, the Virgin Mary, and Sophia.

The first stage, which Jung called Eve, is associated with the earth and fertility. In this stage the anima is almost indistinguishable from the per- sonal mother. The anima is lost in the hidden and dominating power of the man's mother and may have the effect of leaving him with an attachment to her that lasts throughout his life. When the anima remains in this stage, it may seriously impair a man's ability to develop into an adult and have successful relationships with women.

The second stage is a collective and ideal sexual image of woman. While still associated with the sexual act, the woman is individualized and often romanticized. Personified by Helen of Troy, the anima may appear in dreams and fantasies as the seductress.

The third stage of the anima is personified by Mary and gives the capac- ity for lasting relationships and for spiritual connections. This stage raises Eros, erotic love, to the level of devotion.

Sophia, called wisdom in the Bible, is the fourth stage of the develop- ment of the anima. In this stage, she functions as a guide to the man's inner life and helps in his search for meaning.

Application in Homeopathic Practice

The homeopath may now be able to imagine the effects of the anima or animus on homeopathic practice and understand its usefulness in perceiv- ing what needs to be healed in the client. Familiarity with this complex explains why a homeopath of one sex or another must treat some people.

For instance, a woman who is possessed of a strong negative animus may have a great deal of difficulty in being open with a male homeopath, because she projects her negative animus onto him. Conversely, a man who is strongly anima-possessed may project the negative traits of his anima fantasies onto a female homeopath and not be able to express the essence of his suffering.

Those who are strongly possessed by the anima or animus tend to identify with their persona and have a difficult time getting in touch with their true selves. As mentioned before, those identified with the persona often have a masklike face and do not easily move out of the boundaries of this protective covering.

Difficulty in forming relationships is another hint that the anima or animus is an important factor in understanding what needs to be healed in an individual, as is the inability to find one's place in the world. If homeopaths are able to recognize these signs of possession by this archetype, it may serve as a factor in discriminating between remedies, but more importantly, it may help the homeopath judge the length of time that is required for and the difficulties that may be encountered during the healing process. Understanding the nature of anima or animus projection allows for a more realistic evaluation of the state of health.

To return to more familiar territory, the anima and animus can be further understood through a discussion of several well-known homeopathic remedies: *Staphysagria* and *Nux vomica* in terms of the anima of a man, and *Sepia* and *Hyoscyamus* from the perspective of the animus in a woman. Because possession by the anima or animus is so prevalent, almost any indicated remedy may be needed. These examples are given not as a method of prescribing but simply to show how the anima and animus may operate in particular remedy states.

Men who benefit from the homeopathic remedy *Staphysagria* are very often immersed in sexual and romantic fantasies about women. These fantasies may overshadow their ability for intimate relationships. Although they are sensitive and romantic, they tend to attract women who are never able to give them what they need to satisfy their sexual and romantic longing. This is because they are projecting the fantasies onto the women in their life; in other words, it is their anima that is the actual object of their love.

Nux vomica is another remedy that may be indicated in men who are strongly obsessed by the anima in an entirely different way. In this state the man is very sexually attracted to many women, but he is not so concerned with the individual nature of the woman, being only attracted to her on the level of animal sexuality. He often has a great fear and aversion to marriage, but if he does succeed in getting married, he often has affairs with other women. This is an example of possession of an anima that is close to what Jung describes as the first stage of development, in which Eros is developed to the stage at which it is concerned only with the sex urge.

A very important remedy for women who are possessed by the animus is *Sepia*. One of the well-known symptoms of *Sepia* is aversion to sex and aversion to coition. Nevertheless, the woman who needs *Sepia* often has very sexual dreams, especially in the earlier stages in the development of the *Sepia* state. She may also have orgasm during these dreams. She feels irritable in the company of others and prefers to be alone. The woman needing *Sepia* is more in relationship with her inner male, her animus, than she is with her husband, who can never compete for her favors. When her animus is projected outward it creates the irritable, sharp-tongued and quarrelsome state that this remedy is indicated for. The woman is out of tune with her feminine nature, a fact that is exhibited in physical symptoms as well as her mental state. When women have dealt with their shadow and encountered the animus, *Sepia* is often needed as an intercurrent remedy to empower the woman and help her move into her true femininity.

The remedy *Hyoscyamus* is often indicated for a woman when there is possession by an animus that is in the first stages of development. Even when exhibitionistic tendencies and overt sexual overtures are not seen, a woman in this stage has a strong desire for attention that often has sexual overtones. Because she is possessed by an animus that has remained in very early stages, the woman often degrades herself in her relationships to men or is possessed by jealousy. Even if she has attained some degree of development in her intellectual life, she may still be completely subservient to a jealous and dominant animus that projects its reality out into her world.

The encounter with the anima or animus is the pièce de résistance of inner work, allowing one a greater sense of autonomy. Homeopaths have long spoken of increased freedom as one of the indicators of good health. An understanding of the concept of the anima and animus may help homeopaths to understand what is required within the psyche to gain this level of independence. Freeing oneself from the entanglements of the anima or animus and its association with the collective unconscious turns what was once a troublesome foe into a psychological function that can serve as a powerful ally.

Creating an alliance with the anima or animus archetype is a merging of opposites. The outer woman integrates her womanliness with an inner masculinity, and the outer man utilizes the full value of his inner feminine nature. The alchemists often called this merging of opposites the coniunctio, referring to both the combination of chemicals and the spiritual phenomenon of the merging of matter and spirit. Psychologically, the concept of coniunctio is similar, as it refers to a state in which the individual can accept the reality of the paradox of the opposing forces of life. No longer swinging between the opposites of negative and positive, good and evil, love and hate, the individual is able to sustain a middle ground in which the reality is that everything light has a dark side and every hateful act also has the potential for love.

CHAPTER SEVEN

Wholeness

The Archetype of the Self

The actual process of individuation—the conscious coming-to-terms with one's own inner center (psychic nucleus) or Self—generally begins with a wounding of the personality and the suffering that accompanies it. This initial shock amounts to a sort of "call," although it is not often recognized as such.

MARIE-LOUISE VON FRANZ, IN *Man and His Symbols*[1]

The original derivation of the word *health* meant "wholeness," a term with which homeopaths and other holistic practitioners are familiar. *Webster's Revised Unabridged Dictionary* defines *wholeness* as the quality or state of being whole, entire, or sound; entireness; totality, completeness. Through his clinical practice and his study of mythology, spirituality, and indigenous cultures, Jung deduced that the state of wholeness is actually an archetype that helps to lead the individual into a state that transcends egocentricity.

Jung gave this archetype the paradoxical name of "the Self" and described it as something that goes beyond and cannot be contained by the individual. In *Psychology and Alchemy,* he describes it as all encompassing. "The Self is not only the centre, but also the whole circumference which embraces both conscious and unconscious; it is the centre of this totality, just as the ego is the centre of consciousness."[2]

The Self is considered by Jung to be the central archetype that influences all of the archetypal energies, with the purpose of moving an individual toward unity, or what Jung called individuation. This assumes the Self to be a universal ordering force, accessible to human consciousness, that organizes and gives direction to the collective unconscious.

The Self is often portrayed as a king, prophet, or the sun, but the most frequent representation of the Self is the mandala. The term *mandala* is derived from Sanskrit and means "circle" or "magic circle." The mandala appears in the East as a painting or drawing made up of concentrically arranged figures, round or square patterns arranged around a center. The mandala is an attempt on the part of the human mind to visualize the wholeness and vastness of the cosmos while acknowledging the individual pieces that make up the reality of human life. The ultimate purpose of this visualization of the macrocosm is a higher level of psychological or spiritual integration. One of the ways in which spiritual integration is achieved is by meditation on a mandala, which contains many intricate levels leading to a center or godhead. The meditation leads the initiate inward into the depths of his psyche. In their book *Mandala,* Jose and Miriam Arguelles mention a description of this meditation by well-known authority on religion and shamanism, Mircea Eliade:

> As he approaches its center, the disciple approaches the *"center of the world."* In fact, as soon as he has entered the mandala, he is in a sacred space, outside of time; the gods have already "descended." A series of meditations, for which the disciple has been prepared in advance, help him to find the gods in his own heart. In a vision, he sees them all emerge and spring from his heart/ they fill cosmic space, and then are reabsorbed in him. In other worlds, he "realizes" the eternal process of the periodic creation and destruction of the worlds/ and this allows him to enter into the rhythms of the cosmic great time and to understand its emptiness. He shatters the plane of samsara and enters a transcendent plane.[3]

Another method for integrating the wholeness of the mandala is in the act of its creation. The importance of mandalas, such as the Hopi or the Tibetan sand paintings, is in the creation itself, as they are destroyed soon after the process of creation has been completed. Hours and even days can be spent carefully preparing an intricate mandala out of colored sand, only to completely destroy it shortly after it is finished. This lends another facet of human reality to the mandala, impermanence.

Western culture in not without its mandalas. The rose window, a great circle of translucent stained glass, is often an important part of the architecture of the great cathedrals of Christianity. On a sunny day, the sunlight breaks up into multicolored facets, creating the perfect sensual metaphor for multiplicity within unity.

Some mandalas are untouched by human hands but exist in nature, as in a snowflake or in the organization of cellular and atomic life as seen through a microscope. With the development of the electron microscope, the mandala of the order of the universe can now be seen by viewing subatomic particles. These are the mandalas created by nature herself, reflecting the underlying elegant patterning inherent within substance. Is it here, at the point where the ordering factor in human consciousness meets that order within substance, that psyche and substance meet? On the other hand, is the reality that psyche and substance are always connected while we remain blissfully unaware of the fact?

The nature of the Self necessitates investigation of symbols that are connected with various religions, because the existence of the Self is largely a metaphysical question. It is important, however, to differentiate between the symbols as they exist within their religious connotation and the personal experience of the archetype as it appears in dreams and visions of individuals. The archetype of the Self can be better understood through the study of myth and the history of religion. The individual experience is personal. It is an essential point that people may experience the archetype of the Self in their own unique way. For example, an airline pilot may have a dream of the Self in which he is flying his own special flying vehicle. The archetype of the Self may appear as a brilliant gold chest plate to another. It is the individuals association to the symbolism that is of utmost importance.

Dreams are the portal through which we can link directly to the Self and the archetypal realm.

As the powerful ordering factor of nature, the Self is seen and felt through dreams and visions in which mandalas of all types appear as messengers of wholeness. This archetype often appears when there is need for an integrative force to stabilize a traumatic situation. Here, symbolized by the mandala, the Self appears as a beneficent carrier of integrative energy to prevent the disintegration of the personality. Many times this assistance remains in the unconscious, and at other times it reaches consciousness and the dream or vision is remembered for the rest of a person's life.

The mandala can also be seen in dreams of individuals who are about to make or have just made a big step toward wholeness. If the significance of these dreams is understood and consciously integrated, they can profoundly assist in creating that development.

Development of Wholeness

In the process of personal development, there must be development of the ego, a sense of personal self, but in the later part of life, the reverse process challenges an individual. After a person has lived a life identified with the ego, their ego must form a relationship to the archetype of the Self if further development is to take place. Premature aging, ossification of the body and mind, or illness may occur if this process is stymied. Midlife crises and other diseases that occur between forty and fifty are often associated with, among other things, the need to move toward the greater wholeness being exerted upon the individual by the Self.

Some people, especially when they are confronted with a difficult health condition, need to develop the ego and, at the same time, move into wholeness. This requires an interweaving of ego building and integration of the Self, as well as the encounter with the shadow.

The following is the journey of a woman who has gone through this process over a period of several years. As she progresses, she shows a special talent for understanding her dreams and expressing her inner feelings. Her generosity of spirit is shown in her desire to share her healing experience so that it may benefit others.

Linda, a forty-six-year-old psychotherapist, came to homeopathy for alopecia areata, hair loss in patches. The problem had started over two years before, when she lost well over half her hair. She had been treated conventionally with topical steroids that resolved the problem, but the problem then recurred a year later, when her brother died. The hair loss was very upsetting to her. She said, "The hair loss was very disfiguring. In terms of my body—my looks—my hair is of utmost importance." Here is how she described herself and her situation:

> For the last couple of years, I have been trying to meet the reality of living and dying. I have an underlying feeling that I'm doing something wrong and if I stop doing wrong everything will be OK. I'm very sensitive to the suffering of others; their suffering feels real to me. I'm not repulsed by it—I don't go to a place of hardening in my heart.
>
> I'm an incest survivor—I've carried the blame and shame so long—maybe it wouldn't have happened to me if I hadn't done something wrong. I've been trying to survive the self-hatred that I have carried. I didn't know how to have compassion for the little girl who got abused. I blamed her.

In our family you dig in and work hard. Dad always said, "There's nothing you can't do if you work hard enough." As a young child I stayed to myself a lot and read. Rolled down hills. In high school, I became very involved in activities—I can do this kind of thing—get really involved. I felt there was this kind of mission in this. To make up for "being so bad," I'd work hard. In college I was a farm girl who went to the city, was very anxious.

To have needs in my family was to be a burden. I'm one of eight children. I was very good, helpful, hardworking. Didn't want to have anyone say I was a burden. Mom was very distant. She was tired and worn out. I didn't feel known by her. I didn't want to be anything like her—that's why I went to college.

I sometimes feel burned out caring for others. There was confusion about that. Felt that when they were better, it was at my expense. When I am burned out, there is the feeling that no one is there for me, nothing for me, a real regressed place.

I can be very patient. Friends say I'm easy-going, tolerant. Lately, I've been much more irritable. I think a lot, am serious, and can stay really silent. I've had a lot of shame about being shy, but I'm a good worker and supporter. I think it has to do with my shyness.

There's a way that I disconnect from others and myself. I disassociate and get involved with compulsive working. It's a way that I've held onto a kind of judgment about myself.

The second time she lost her hair, she had a dream. She said the dream was "about the book of wisdom. It's about how it is important not to test God. To allow faith to bring you to a place of trust. When you test God—it's turning away. So the challenge is to be more trusting."

Based on the hair loss, timid personality, her confusion about the abuse, and the fact that she spoke very slowly and seemed confused, she was given the homeopathic remedy *Alumina*. Because she was very concerned about losing any more hair, an LM potency, which is a very dilute but not highly succussed homeopathic preparation, was used to avoid aggravation of her symptoms. The LM potency of *Alumina* was continued in ascending potency throughout this period of her treatment.

The need for *Alumina* is frequently difficult to see, because patients who need this remedy often lack symptoms on which to prescribe. They often have a certain vagueness and confusion in the way they relate to themselves and their situation. *Alumina* is one of the main remedies when there is confusion of identity—lack of ego development.

The ego is connected with the conscious, individual part of the person. It is about uniqueness, the sense of being an individual separate and unique from others. When a person has very little sense of who they are, it is because the ego has not fully developed, as it should in early life. This is frequently the case in persons who have not had a nurturing family life.

Not only is it important for the ego to be developed, but the ego must also have flexibility and resilience for it to be connected to the Self. Because the Self contains all opposites and is accepting of all opposites, connection with this wholeness gives the individual an underlying feeling of acceptance. No matter what the individual's action, the Self has the capacity to reconcile all opposites. Otherwise, any activity in life can throw the ego back and forth within the play of opposites like a boat without a captain. This connection or communication between the Self and the ego is what the late Jungian analyst Edward Edinger calls the ego-Self axis. He describes it as "the vital connecting link between ego and Self that ensures the integrity of the ego."[4]

Infants are totally identified with the Self, and their sense of individuality, which is realized through the development of the ego, is developed later. This is done through projection onto the parents, especially the mother, as the child grows older. In this time of projection, the ego-Self axis is very vulnerable to damage. The parenting must consist of just the right amount of support for the development of the child as an individual. If the parent is too lax in setting boundaries and rules, the child will grow up thinking that they are the center of the universe. The ego will become inflated to such an extent that the individual ego identifies with the Self. On the other hand, if the parent is too strict, ignores, or abuses the child, the connection to the Self is damaged.

The individual who needs *Alumina* is often dealing with severe damage to the ego-Self axis from actual or perceived trauma in early childhood. These individuals are like the character of Estelle in Sartre's *No Exit*, who wonders if she exists at all if she cannot see her reflection in a mirror. In the *Alumina* state, the individual knows he or she exists only through projection.

As in Linda's case, many people who have lost connection with the Self through childhood trauma have done many therapies or are therapists themselves, but the wound has not been healed. Because the wound occurred at a very early, perhaps preverbal stage, it is difficult to access the problem through mental and emotional symptoms. When there are physical symptoms that lead to the correct homeopathic remedy, homeopathy may be able to help these people.

If the homeopath also understands the role the psyche plays in the healing process, there is an even better chance that the individual will be able to move into a new level of health and wholeness.

One month after taking the remedy, Linda reported that her hair had stopped falling out and was growing back. She had also begun to reflect on how she had developed patterns to skirt around her confusion. Through her reflections, she allowed herself to go into the confusion and make it clearer. In other words, at that point in her therapy, she had the ego strength to allow herself to see how confused she had been.

During the first month of taking the remedy, she had the following dream. "There were all these babies (five of them). I was in charge of feeding them, and I fed them nipple to nipple."

When questioned about the dream, she replied, "I feel that this remedy is working from a very young age. In the dream it was so *easy,* plenty of milk. No burden. Working with the heart."

Her specific association to the nipples was that, "I just plugged into them, into that place of suckling, of life force energy. The place of figuring out doesn't work. It's the opening and flowing. Safety is within me. Not depending on the outside."

This was an initial dream, a dream that predicted something of the outcome of the therapy. It predicted that she has the possibility to reconnect to the Self. The dream created a striking metaphor of what it is like for her to relate to the Self; she "just plugs in" to that nourishing energy—the life force. As she said, safety is within her and she does not need to depend on the outside. This is what it is like, ultimately, for the ego to connect with a reality bigger than itself.

In her dream, there were five babies. Five is the quinary in alchemy, the number of created being and individuality (Self and ego). The dream maker within the psyche was speaking a language that the therapist could understand. The psyche seeks help wherever it can get it.

Linda had done a lot of healing work previous to homeopathic treatment, but the connection to the Self was still damaged. We see from the dream that the remedy was working, or would work, very deeply. It was repairing the ego-Self axis. The dream showed that this had either happened already or would happen in the future. With this assurance, the homeopath proceeded with the same remedy, but in a higher level of potency.

After two months, Linda's hair continued to grow in, and she no longer had the feeling of having done something wrong. She began to get even more information from her dreams and felt that they were helping her understand herself. She reported two dreams. The first dream was about zombies. "I'm outside. Zombies are in the trees; wasn't sure if I should be afraid. I wasn't sure what zombies did."

She felt that the zombies were symbols of the dead parts of her, parts that her family taught her must be dead. She said, "They stand for what was dead in me. In my family we were taught not to go outside the family. That the world is dangerous. That constricts me." The remedy and the dream analysis were bringing these dead parts of her to the conscious level.

This deadness, sometimes described as robot-like behavior, is a symptom often seen in those who need the remedy *Alumina*. Often the people speak of themselves in the third person, as if they weren't present. This deadness was there, according to Linda's association to the dream, because she was taught by her family to be this way. Her dreams also showed a connection to the sexual abuse, because she presented a second dream that relates to this abuse. Dreams that are dreamt in the same night or those that are reported together, as she reported these two dreams, are usually connected.

Her second dream was about the man who sexually abused her when she was a child. "My uncle had a razor blade, and he was coming to kill me. I knew I could call 911 and get help, and I didn't have to go to where it was unsafe."

Here, she revisited the horror of the early childhood abuse, but this time the perpetrator couldn't harm her, because she had become more conscious and had developed the ability to react. The second dream followed, after she had become aware of the zombie parts of her psyche. In bringing awareness to them, she was now able to replay the abuse in a different way. This is a wonderful dream of revisiting and healing the trauma. It shows the healing capacity within the psyche. The homeopath continued Linda on the same remedy.

Up until that point in therapy, Linda had been feeling much better, but she began to have more intense feelings, including negative feelings that she had never allowed herself to experience. She had periods of despair. Her shadow was beginning to emerge. At her fourth month of homeopathic treatment, she said that she was horrified by the following dream that she had a week prior to her consultation: "There was a group of people sitting around a table and a man was doing a demo on how to use a pistol—to show them how to put it to their heads and kill themselves."

It is very important to let people know that they can dream anything they want and they will not be judged for it. The nicer a person is in daily life, the more horrible his or her dreams may be. St. Augustine thanked God for not making him responsible for his dreams. Since dreams often compensate for the waking state, it is understandable that a saint would probably have very unsaintly dreams.

Linda's association to this dream was that it was about "a pattern of self-destructiveness that I'm trying to put to an end." When asked about the group she replied:

> *The group is my family. It is the group thinking that I took in from my family. It's mindless groupthink. Even now, I had this knowing that the dream was good—but I always play dumb because I need to play down my own power. I'm always apologizing for my own opinions.*

Although she hesitated at first because of the violence of the dream, and a fear that she would be judged for having it, she knew exactly what the dream was about; she was killing parts of her psyche that were identified with the "groupthink" of her family. She had previously lost her own identity to the beliefs and attitudes of her family members. This is something that those needing *Alumina* are particularly prone to do. They easily identify with the group and lose their individual identity to the group identity. This may be the meaning of one symptom found in the provings of this remedy: "fear of knives for fear that she may kill someone." Perhaps a psychic need is being expressed through this symptom.

Linda was now in the process of creating her own sense of self and was very clear about the meaning of the dream. On the other hand, she was still afraid to express herself. As she said, "I'm always apologizing for my own opinions."

After her fifth month of treatment her hair was much thicker than it had been, but she still had one small spot of hair loss. She said that she had much better clarity of mind and had been handling conflicts with others much better.

After hearing on the news of an airline flight that crashed and killed all the passengers, she had the following dream:

> *I was walking through a dense forest—sunlight was filtering through the trees. I came to a clearing and saw all the people who had been on that flight, strapped into their seats. They were all dead. I had the sense*

*that I had to pray for them—the Hail Mary. I had to pray for them
because they were so confused from the trauma.*

When asked about her association with the dream she replied, "Since the
remedy—all these dead things have been in my dreams—they were trapped in
the confusion of my trauma. What is needed now is prayer and surrender."Her
association to the Hail Mary prayer was that it was about the "trust that—
now and at the hour of our death—there is someone. It is a way of not being
alone."

Mary, she said, is "the mother who is really there—she is a way of connecting through and with the mother. It was a beautiful dream; I needed to
pray the next day. I wasn't frightened at all."

Because Mary is an archetype of the mother, the homeopath encouraged
a discussion about the meaning of Mary on this level. Linda said that there
was a relationship between her mother, herself, and Mary: "This is a connection I share with my mother—my mother loves the rosary and loves
Mary. She once said when she was ill, 'Mary shows me that I'm not alone.'"
Linda believed the dream meant that it was time for prayer and surrender.
The prayer was the Hail Mary. Mary, who in Christianity is the mother of
god, is the archetype of the mother. Because the archetypes are found in the
collective unconscious, this meant that, at least in this dream, Linda was
moving into a realm of her psyche that connects with a larger reality than
her own personal unconscious and her ego.

Moving into this realm, she connected with her own birth mother through
the archetype. Many times this is how traumatic relationships with parents
can be healed. A loving relationship can be developed with parents who are
indifferent, cruel, or incapable of relationship through contact with the
archetypal energies of mother and father.

Contact with the mother archetype, because it is associated with physical
matter and earthly existence, also brings with it connection to the world
and specifically to the body. This is particularly important when severe
trauma has led to disassociation from the body.

After six months Linda was not so concerned about her hair—it was fine.
She had a dream about a violent man.

*I took the car in for repair, but I could see it was steaming while at
a traffic light. At the shop there was an exotic macho mechanic who was
showing his boss a picture of two men. He said he had killed them with
a curved knife. Once he disemboweled someone.*

I was aware of how frightened I was—but I gave him the car. Then when I get the car back it's not fixed. I woke up with a dilemma—how am I going to confront him with this.

Linda knew by this point in therapy that a dream like this more often represented the inner workings of her own psyche. She associated the mechanic in the dream, who had disemboweled someone, to her own tendency to slice herself up with rough expectations. One could also say that this man represented her animus, her inner male. He was the one who beats her up all the time.

She began to understand this as she connected the fact that he was exotic and macho with male dominance, violence, use of power, and mystery. These are qualities of her animus. Some of these qualities are very negative, but if she could confront her animus, she would acquire some of his intensity. The fact that the man in her dream was associated with mystery pointed to the fact that her animus was still in the shadow, mostly unknown and unconscious.

However, it looked like she already had been affected by the confrontation with the animus. She said that the car steaming up represented her anger. She had been very angry with her husband. The steaming up, or anger, led her to bring her car to the mechanic/animus. The animus archetype had become activated, and of course, she projected it onto her husband.

She associated her car with something that was important to her, something she depended on. She had left this important thing with this scary man with a knife, and he hadn't fixed the car. She woke up with the thought, "How am I going to confront him about this?" How indeed. Confrontation of the animus is no easy matter.

After working with this first dream she remembered another one.

I was in a boat with a baby who was fully grown—like a tiny adult in a fetal position. It felt ancient, like a totem, and we're trying to take this baby somewhere.

Just as a totem is a symbol of something to be treated with respect, it is sometimes important to allow a dream's mystery to unfold without trying try to understand it. This was one of those dreams, and it may have been saying how the confrontation with the animus would be resolved.

Her dreams began to make more sense as they followed one another and it became possible to get an idea of the intelligence behind the process. For the next year, Linda continued her homeopathic treatment. She was, in her words, "having a rich but difficult time."

At a certain point, she had gotten in touch with a lot of hatred that had come up from "a very young place." She said she had had "to ride a wave of self-hatred that was covering over deeper pain." She had been preparing herself to feel this. "In this dark place," she said, "I couldn't find God—but there was a knowing of its existence."

This is the "dark night of the soul," or *nigredo*, that necessarily follows a confrontation with the archetypal contents of the psyche. For Linda, this feeling lasted for a few months and then cleared up. She felt very well and was excited about what was going on in her life. She said, "I know that part of my wounding was that I had to stay small. Now I'm moving out. That creates fear—but not fear that will annihilate me. My work with clients is exciting. The space we enter together is deeper and deeper. Effortless but with effort. My relationship to my ego is different. I know that I am more than my ego."

At that point, she had a dream that she understood very well:

> *My family and I were traveling in an open boxcar. We hit a bump, and my mother-in-law was catapulted out. I got out and went down the path. She had landed in a wheelchair and was fine. Her mouth and arms were bound, and I was going to unbind her.*

Her analysis of the dream was that she was healing generations of women who were bound. This indicated that she had been able to integrate the animus to such an extent that she was able to release the binding effects of the negative animus on a collective level. This in turn enabled her to experience a deep connection with the Self.

She had been writing poetry and, during that time, wrote a poem about her experience over the year and a half she spent in treatment. Her poem describes the process with great clarity.

Splendor/Victory

How could I have known
That the victory I learned
Was not true victory?

Generations through generations
Have tried to conquer people and their land.

There is no splendor that comes from annihilation.
Mistakes are denied because no value of self exists.

Only through the victory of honesty
Have I begun to come into relationship with
My own cruelty and my own hatred.
Simultaneously a larger view of how heaven includes
        hell exists.
Choice from place emerges, freedom reigns.

Give thanks to the Lord our God
Whose mercy endures forever.[5]

Descent into the Bath
Moving Toward the Union of the Opposites

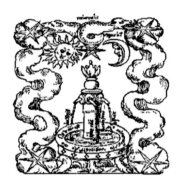

As a part of their laboratory work, the alchemists would often put silver and gold together in a bath of mercury, in order to form an amalgam. Formation of an amalgam is also part of the process of inner alchemy and is shown in old woodcuts as a king and a queen entering into a bath. These images can be seen as the opposing forces within the mind-body that are in need of unification.

After the parts of the psyche have been defined, it is possible to descend into the world of the psyche through the process of dream analysis. This third section will cover the use of dreams in early medicine and how dream imagery relates to the mind-body. How to ask about dreams and the way in which the psyche of the homeopath affects dream work will be investigated, and there will be a chapter on the subtle technique of dream analysis.

CHAPTER EIGHT

Dreams and the Mind-Body Relationship
The Use of Dreams in Homeopathic Practice

With a brief outline of homeopathy and concepts of Jungian thought, it is now possible to discuss integrating the use of dreams and symbolism into homeopathic practice. The wisdom of the ancients, combined with Jung's study of the unconscious, can help the practitioner understand the nature of what needs to be healed and what is required to stimulate that healing.

Homeopaths have used dreams since Hahnemann's time. Our repertories and provings contain many references to dreams, yet many questions remain about how to use dreams effectively in homeopathic practice.

One huge change that has taken place since Hahnemann's time has been the birth of the field of psychology and the development of our understanding of the unconscious. Although Hahnemann was ahead of his time in the treatment of mental illness, very little understanding of what came to be called the psyche was available to him. Most studies of the mind were limited to the physiology of the brain and various theories about how the mind might actually work.

Franz Anton Mesmer (1734-1815), a contemporary of Hahnemann, was a controversial German physician who developed methods of hands-on healing and hypnotherapy (the term *mesmerized* derived from his practices). He recognized the role that the mind played in disease. Although Hahnemann thought very highly of Mesmer's work, which he called "a wonderful, priceless gift of God, granted to humanity," he interpreted mesmerism as transmission of the mesmerist's life force to the patient.[1]

It was not until several years after Hahnemann's death that Freud developed his seminal works on psychotherapy, the unconscious, and dream analysis.

The rationalist ideas of the eighteenth-century Age of Reason caused medical practitioners, along with people in other professions, to regard the wisdom from the past as superstition. And so, while dreams have had a role in medicine for thousands of years, very little medical use of dreams survived into the early nineteenth century.

In a way, dreams have never had a more important potential role in homeopathic case taking than they have in the present era. When homeopaths in earlier times asked about food desires, physical modalities, and sensations, they could usually depend on clear, straightforward answers. Today, it is rare to find individuals who have not had most of their mental, general, and physical symptoms suppressed. We now live in a very complex and overmedicated society that is reluctant to allow any symptom to go untreated or untrained—or to allow any desire to go uncensored and uninfluenced by advertising and media. Most people live a life that is so removed from nature that symptoms become intellectualized and therefore unreliable, making it very difficult to picture who the individual really is. Fortunately, dreams lie outside our conscious ability to manipulate them. We cannot create a false reality in our dreams or influence them with our will. Material that is suppressed from the conscious state moves into the subconscious and is frequently expressed in dreams. Because the dream is a deep expression of the workings of the psyche, material from dreams, when used and analyzed accurately, can lead to some of the most reliable symptoms in a case. Although they seem ephemeral, dreams are actually objective facts about a person's mental and physical state.

Carl Jung said that there was most likely no difference between body and mind. Rather, they are what he called "the same life," subject to the same laws. What happens in the body is reflected in the mind, and vice versa. Dreams are proof that this unbreakable connection still exists, even though we often operate under the delusion that the mind and body are separate.

All homeopaths are aware of the connection between mind and body—although using a dream as if it were a separate symptom and not an integral part of the entire case misses the importance of this connection. Because homeopathic practice was formed before the understanding of the relationship between the body and psyche was fully developed, dreams are often used without a deep understanding of their true role in the case.

Exploring the messages the unconscious sends in the dream state will help us use dreams to enrich what is commonly called the "red thread that runs throughout the case." It is also possible to get a clear picture of pathology from a dream, and to use symbolic information from the dream state to understand the process that is about to unfold.

Dreams are also our primary connection to the inherited wisdom of the psyche. They help us reconnect with a level that has been largely ignored in rationally focused Western societies and afford an opportunity to integrate the symbolic with the rational.

For millennia, the symbolic world ruled: ultimately; it overwhelmed the individual and society, causing them to fall prey to fear and superstition. The Enlightenment, with its more rational, mind-centered view of the world, was a necessary corrective, a vital evolutionary step; now, however, humanity's move toward the rational has developed into a technical and scientific world that has all but obscured the connection to the symbolic realm. Another evolutionary step is now needed—the integration of the rational and the symbolic. The symbolic language of dreams allows us to go beyond our limited and contained view of reality and move into a more universal and expanded understanding, giving us access to connections that would be difficult or impossible to make through rational thought.

Rational thought, as useful and necessary as it is, remains ego bound and, as such, does not allow for the unknown. It tends to tie itself up in its own concepts. Jung, who devoted his life to studying the imagery of the psyche, used dreams as a primary method of investigation and felt that dreams were one of the most important ways of understanding the deepest aspect of an individual. In the following passage from *Civilization in Transition*, he speaks of the dream as a portal to a more universal reality:

> *A dream is a little hidden door in the deepest and most intimate sanctum of the soul, which opens into that primeval cosmic night that was psyche long before there was any ego-consciousness and which will remain psyche no matter how far our ego-consciousness extends. For all ego-consciousness is isolated; because it separates and discriminates, it knows only particulars, and it sees only those that can be related to the ego. Its essence is limitation, even though it reach to the farthest nebulae among the stars. All consciousness separates; but in dreams we put on the likeness of that more universal, truer, more eternal man dwelling in the darkness of primordial night.*[2]

Dreams appear as images, which are a more primary way of thinking than language. In addition, these images are often symbols. A symbol is an image that points to a larger picture: it is an experience that extends beyond itself to a greater reality than can be reached through the limitation of human thought. Although a symbol is filtered through human consciousness and is therefore only partly valid, it is still the best possible expression of the mystery that it attempts to describe.

Healers who live in touch with the mystery of the symbolic world in its purest form have traditionally been called shamans. They have existed in all times and places, and continue to exist today. A look at their experience reveals that many of the symbols shamans encounter also exist in the myths of cultures far removed from them and, indeed, in the dreams of city dwellers today.

Shamanism: Lifting the Veil to the Mystery of Symbolism

With their deep and rich contact with the symbolic realm, the experiences of shamans offer another way, besides dream work, of entering into the mystery of symbolism. The role of the shaman emerged from humans' earliest experience with symbols. Shamans were individuals who could communicate directly with the gods and act as intermediaries for the general population, to supplicate the gods and help the community prepare itself to face the overwhelming power of the forces of nature. One of the prized abilities of the shaman was the ability to understand symbols and to interpret dreams. Most shamans were initiated into their practice by their own illness, and through symbolic knowledge received in dreams or visions. Often, through these initiatory dreams, the shaman learned how to cure illness—their own illnesses and ultimately all similar illnesses—even receiving explicit information on specific treatments for particular diseases. The following is an account of the experience of initiation of a Samoyed shaman, from Siberia, who had been sick with smallpox and was almost dying.

> *He remembered having been carried into the middle of a sea. There he heard his Sickness speak, saying to him: From the Lords of the Water you will receive the gift of shamanizing. Your name as a shaman will be Houtataire (Diver). Then the Sickness troubled the water of the sea. The candidate came out and climbed a mountain. There he met a naked woman and began to suckle at her breast. The woman, who was probably the Lady of the Water, said to him: "You are my child; that is why I let you suckle at my breast. You will meet many hardships and be greatly wearied." The husband of the Lady of the Water, the Lord of the*

Underworld, then gave him two guides, an ermine and a mouse, to lead him to the underworld. When they came to a high place, the guides showed him seven tents with torn roofs. He entered the first and there found the inhabitants of the underworld and the men of the Great Sickness (syphilis). These men tore out his heart and threw it into a pot. In other tents he met the Lord of Madness and the Lords of all the nervous disorders, as well as the evil shamans. Thus he learned the various diseases that torment mankind.[3]

The vision goes on to introduce the shaman to the powers contained in the animal and plant world, finally introducing him to the spirits of the mountains. One of the interesting aspects of this vision is that it contains many universal or archetypal symbols that have remained much the same for thousands of years and have an astounding similarity from culture to culture and epoch to epoch. When these images appear in dreams and visions, they relate not only to the individual dreamer but also to a more universal knowledge which, to use the Jungian term, we may call the collective unconscious. While archetypes may be colored by individual or cultural beliefs, they are primordial impulses of life. These dreams are larger than the dreamer. They speak not only to the needs of the individual but also to the needs of the time.

The Lady of the Water who calls the shaman her child and lets him suckle is one such universal symbol; it appears in many times and many cultures. There is a fifteenth-century woodcut by the alchemist Mylius that is remarkably similar to the scene described by this Siberian shaman. In it, the Earth suckles the *filius philosophorum,* or "divine child."

This theme appears over and over again in dreams, visions, and spiritual literature. The image here represents the archetype of Gaia, the Earth Mother. Archetypes such as this are much more than individual consciousness and are not limited to specific cultures or eras. True, they will be colored by individual or cultural beliefs, but the underlying motif is the same. These archetypes are primordial impulses of life and as such are influenced by, but not made up entirely of, human consciousness. In the initiation of the shaman, the Earth Mother comes to show him how to help humanity. The Earth Mother of the alchemists shows her supporting the *filius philosophorum,* or "divine child," representing the potential for wholeness which is the hoped-for outcome of the alchemists' art.

The Samoyed shaman's dream experience shows that the unconscious is not only filled with dangerous and terrible things, as some may fear. The vast sphere of the psyche contains as much that helps as there is to hinder. Individual life is so fragile that without a stable connection to a deeper reality we are blown about in the wind. One of the methods to alleviate the fear and suffering inherent within this fragile isolation is to admit our weakness and call on help from within.

Dreams in Early Medicine

Throughout history, physicians, as well as shamans, have used dreams to aid them in diagnosis and treatment of disease. Dreams have played an important role in Eastern medicine for thousands of years and still do, because many of these forms of medicine have remained in their original state and have not succumbed to the mechanistic view of the body and mind.

The Yellow Emperor's Classic of Internal Medicine (2696 B.C.), a text on Chinese medicine believed to be the oldest medical book still in existence, contains a section devoted to dreams and their relationship to illness. Certain dreams were said to indicate the flow and type of energy in the body. Dreams of sorrow and weeping were thought to indicate problems in the lungs, and dreams of great fires were said to indicate a flourishing of yang energy.

Ayurveda, an ancient form of medicine originating in India, utilizes dreams to help differentiate between the three types of people and disease—kapha, pitta, and vata—and the interpretation of dreams is an important part of the Ayurvedic medical interview. Those with a kapha constitution or condition are said to have romantic dreams, often of lakes or ponds, and those with a pitta imbalance will have violent dreams, including dreams of war. Those needing treatment for vata imbalance may have fearful dreams.

In Tibetan medicine, a system that looks upon the patient as a precious human being, the interpretation of dreams has always been an essential part of diagnosis and prognosis. Ancient medical texts describe the major categories of dreams, including those arising from illness and dreams predicting illness and death. Because Tibetan physicians are concerned with the quality of life as well as the treatment of disease, they examine the dreams of both healthy and sick people. These practitioners, who talk to and keenly observe the patient, take the pulse, examine the urine, and listen to dreams before giving a diagnosis. The ability of some Tibetan physicians to pinpoint the cause of a patient's symptoms using these techniques has astonished Western physicians who have observed the procedure. If the dreams and other signs indicate illness, dietary changes, meditation, and breathing exercises may be prescribed, as well as medications. If dreams and other signs foretell death, the physician will tell family members, who are then instructed in how to prepare for the patient's death. Only if the patient is very strong and able to cope with the information will the physician tell the patient of the prediction

Dream incubation, the ritual of acknowledging and giving great value to dreams for the purpose of healing, is thought to have first been used by ancient Egyptian physicians. The incubation ritual gave power and influence to dreams, which were thought to be messages from the gods. The ancient Egyptians, and later the Greeks, saw sickness as the result of divine action to be cured by a god or other divine action—an application of the homeopathic principle of the law of similars.

The dreams were interpreted in three different ways, depending on the era and upon the dream itself. The first way of perceiving a dream from an incubation ritual was that the dream itself represented the manifestation of healing from the gods. In these cases, no further treatment was needed, as the dream itself was the cure. This view of dreams relied on the self-healing capacity of the psyche, a reality that can often be observed through following the development of an individual in many forms of therapy. The second way was to see the dream as giving direct information to the physician as to what medication, lifestyle change, or diet was necessary. The third method of utilizing the dream was for the physician to interpret the symbols in dreams in a more routine way.

Imhotep, a legendary and multifaceted Egyptian physician who lived in the twenty-seventh century B.C., designed the famous Step Pyramid of Djoser and developed a form of medicine based on information revealed in his patients' dreams. Surrounding the Step Pyramid were temples of healing where people would come to special chambers for dream incubation. Modern visitors to the Step Pyramid and its complex of buildings can still experience the grand entrance room, with its refreshing pool where patients prepared themselves, before being ushered into small rooms created especially for dream incubation. In the rooms, the patients would sleep and await prophetic or healing dreams that were then interpreted by the priest/physicians of the temple, who would prescribe remedies based on the dreams' symbolism.

Egyptian dream incubation had an influence on Greek physicians, and many ancient Greek temples were devoted to Aesculapius, the god of healing and medicine, who was said to appear in dreams to bestow healing. One of the most famous of these temples was the Aesclepion, on Kos, the island that was the birthplace of Hippocrates. These temples were dedicated, among other things, to healing and dreaming. People entering the Aesclepion had to fast and cleanse themselves. Then they slept in a special chamber in which they would receive a healing dream. This dream could be healing in itself—it could include the healing touch of a god—or it could give symbolic information that the Hippocratic physician would interpret as indicating a particular herb, unguent, or other treatment.

The fourth book of the Hippocratic work *On Regimen in Acute Diseases* describes dreams that predict physiological problems. This work includes an explanation of their causes, with suggested interpretations of their meaning. Plato wrote in his *Republic* that dreams revealed the inner passions of the dreamer, and his student Aristotle believed that dreams were sensitive indicators of bodily conditions that could predict illness.

The Greek physician Galen (A.D. 130–200), in his treatise *On Diagnosis from Dreams*, gives dreams medical interpretations: Someone dreaming of smoke, mist, or deep darkness, for example, is bothered by black bile. Aside from *On Regimen in Acute Diseases* and *On Diagnosis from Dreams*, most Hippocratic physicians were not concerned if the dreams were messengers from the gods; rather, the physicians used dreams as a diagnostic and prognostic tool, without trying to explain why those dreams reflected physical conditions. Dreams were another part of the information that the patient brought forth in order to perceive what needed to be cured and to choose an appropriate therapy.

Dreams and Symbols as Early Warnings of Disease

It is now known that chronic diseases have their onset many years before symptoms appear. Symptoms of arteriosclerosis have been found in the bodies of healthy young men who have been killed in accidents or in wartime. It is estimated that this disease may begin as early as the age of four. Because the psyche has knowledge of the state of the body, one avenue for detecting very early stages of bodily imbalance is through dreams and the symbolic language of the psyche.

Dreams and symbols can be used to tap into intuitive logic. Their symbolic messages give insight into an order that lies beyond not only the reach of the intellect but even beyond the ability of advanced diagnostic procedures.

When complemented by technological advances in medicine that allow for concrete evaluation, dream analysis allows the therapist to use the organizing principle within the collective unconscious to reveal important facts about the disharmony within the mind-body complex.

The symbolic language of the psyche communicates through emotional and bodily symptoms, pains and dysfunctions, as well as through dreams, and the messages in dreams and the physical distresses of an individual are often connected. This connection enriches the symbolic metaphor of the disharmony.

Kate was in her forties when she appeared for homeopathic treatment to help with hot flashes, extreme sensitivity to heat, and high blood pressure. She had a history of headaches and was overweight. On the emotional level, she had a very strong desire to contain her emotions and rarely lost her temper or felt angry. She studied many self-help techniques that helped her to maintain a positive attitude. These techniques helped her contain her anger and other emotions that she perceived as being negative. She also complained of a pervasive feeling of loneliness.

Kate had a recurring dream since childhood that the house would catch on fire. She also had a fear of fire from an early age. When questioned as to what this meant to her, she spoke not of the fire itself but of a fear that the stove in the house would explode. Her dreams and fears were giving her a symbolic message from an early age. This message began long before she developed physical symptoms.

Her physical symptoms of high blood pressure, sensitivity to heat, and headaches all relate to the early symbolic message. She had always bottled up her emotions and never lost her temper—hence fear of explosion—and now her body was building up pressure under the strain. The increase in blood pressure could possibly lead to a very dangerous problem related to explosion—a cardiovascular accident, which is, of course, a form of explosion.

The homeopathic remedy that was able to help Kate was likewise made from an extremely explosive substance—*Nitroglycerine,* or *Glonoinum,* a remedy that has been used by homeopaths for over a hundred years. This remedy, along with proper conventional medication, was able to bring balance to Kate's most serious problem, to the point that her physician gave her a clean bill of health.

The relationship between Kate's physical problems and the symbolic messages from her psyche clearly shows that successful treatment had to address her underlying psychic state. Her psyche had been communicating symbolically since her childhood, clearly describing the disease state that had been developing from a very early age.

The symbolism from the dream of fire and the physical symptoms led to an understanding of the imbalance that had existed from childhood. Fire is one of those archetypal symbols that make up the collective unconscious. People who have a strong connection with this archetype have unique challenges in their lives. Jung writes the following paragraph about those who have a special connection with this archetype:

> As bringers of light, that is, enlargers of consciousness, they overcome darkness, which is to say that they overcome the earlier unconscious state. Higher consciousness, or knowledge going beyond our present day consciousness, is equivalent to being all alone in the world. This loneliness expresses the conflict between the bearer or symbol of higher consciousness and his surroundings. The conquerors of darkness go far back into primeval times, and together with many other legends, prove that there once existed a state of original psychic distress, namely unconsciousness.[4]

The knowledge of an individual archetype, or what Jung described as the archetypal core of an individual complex, helps the therapist to more fully understand the challenges and potentials of the patient. To be connected with the archetype of fire is to be a bringer of light to the world and to consequently feel the isolation inherent within that state. It is the difficult challenge of many creative artists and pioneers. But, no matter how difficult, the path must be pursued, for if this powerful energy is not utilized, it can easily turn against the individual, causing not only physical disease but neurosis as well.

Jung spoke of neurosis as unrealized creative potential, which, when not utilized, is psychic energy that turns into poison. This poison can destroy the health and well-being of the individual and interferes with his or her relationships with others. Those with unlived creativity feel so dissatisfied that they may even attempt to destroy the creativity of others around them.

Given all of this, we could say that the true "cure" for Kate is to achieve her potential in life—to be able to express the fiery aspect of herself in an integrated and meaningful way, to bring her light into the world in a way that increases not only her consciousness but also the consciousness of others.

The Dream as Compensation for the Conscious State

Dreams can often show what an individual needs to compensate for in his or her conscious state. In other words, the dream may show the exact opposite of an individual's waking state. When St. Augustine once thanked God for not making him responsible for his dreams, he could well have been thinking of those dreams that were the opposite of—and compensations for—his saintly life. We can only imagine what the specific content of those dreams must have been. Conversely, people who continually commit evil acts in their waking lives often have very sweet and loving dreams.

In the consulting room, a dream may show the therapist the state that is the direct opposite of what the individual is experiencing in life. One must ask if there is something missing in the individual or if there is some behavior in the waking state that needs the kind of compensation a dream can offer. We can suspect that compensation is at work when the same theme repeats itself again and again in dreams. For example, a man who continually dreams of being at a huge feast where he can eat whatever he wants may be missing out on the "feast of life" in his daily activities. People suffering from chronic depression often have dreams of this sort, in which the individual derives no satisfaction from the usual sensual pleasures of life. Of course, the interpretation of the dream would be different for different people, depending upon their associations to the symbolism in the dream and the circumstances of their lives. No dream is therapeutically meaningful alone and outside of the context of the dreamer.

Fantasies and delusions may, for the purpose of discovering compensation as well as other symbolic meanings, be treated in the same way as dreams. "Building air castles," a symptom often found in those who require the homeopathic remedy *China officinalis,* is an example of compensation appearing in a kind of waking dream: The mind creates great accomplishments in compensation for the lack of accomplishment in reality. If *China officinalis* is the appropriate remedy, it will eventually improve the individual's confidence and satisfaction with life, and the psyche will no longer need to create "air castles" to compensate for the dissatisfaction.

It can even be said that all of a person's history can be viewed as a waking dream that is projected out from the unconscious and onto the body and outside environment. It is a dream that must often be shattered if the individual is to move to a state of greater health.

Symbolic Communication Between Psyche and Body

We have already seen that the psyche can express itself through the body with physical symptoms and the body can communicate through the psyche in dreams. Sometimes, a dream is told at the beginning of treatment that the practitioner familiar with dreams may perceive as divulging the entire imprint of the patient's life, including diagnosis and prognosis of disease. Jung mentions such a dream, told to him by a seventeen-year-old girl who was suspected to be in the first stages of progressive muscular atrophy. Jung was able to analyze the dream and to understand through his analysis that the patient had a terminal illness.[5]

The body can also give messages as to the state of the mind. Freud recognized that neurotic symptoms—hysteria, certain types of pain, and abnormal behavior—are symbolically meaningful. These symptoms are the way that the psyche expresses itself through the body. An example would be the development of throat spasms whenever the patient tries to swallow food when confronted with a situation that the patient finds intolerable and "just can't swallow," or the appearance of paralysis of the legs in someone who "just can't go on" anymore.

The symbolic language of the psyche and body is an attempt by deeper levels of the psyche to communicate important information about health and well-being. Therefore, no medical professional, can afford to ignore the realm of dreams and symbolism

Because homeopathic philosophy has always recognized that the mind and body are not separate but intertwined and homeopathic remedies address both mind and body, homeopathy is able to utilize these symbolic messages more easily than most forms of treatment. Symbolic messages can be used to more fully understand what needs to be cured, to follow the process of healing, and to determine the next course of treatment.

Experienced and well-trained homeopaths follow guidelines that are essential in understanding the patient's progress toward health. These guidelines include understanding the nature of individual reaction to a remedy, the need for the body to cleanse itself of the disease, and the movement of disease from deeper to more superficial levels.

Dreams can add to this knowledge by speaking directly to the matter. They can be useful in determining the efficacy of the remedy and can point toward the need for a second prescription. This help is especially useful when the individual is taking other medications, which may mask many of the symptoms.

A case in point is the dream of a woman who was treated quite successfully with homeopathy over a period of years. After a good response to the same remedy over time, the remedy stopped working, and she had the following dream: "I went out into my garden, and I saw some flowers blooming—up close the foliage was black and unhealthy. The soil was too boggy. There was a need to bring in new soil and help with drainage."

This dream was a hint to the homeopath about the need for a new remedy. The term *soil* is often used in homeopathy to refer to the terrain, or the inherited basis of disease—in other words, the miasmatic level. The inherited basis of disease is frequently treated with remedies that address this issue when the original remedy stops working. The use of these remedies is sometimes referred to as *"drainage."* The symbolism in this dream, along with her physical symptoms, indicated the need for the remedy *Psorinum.* This remedy cleansed the "soil" or inherited tendency toward disease, raised her energy, and subsequently allowed the original remedy to continue to work.

Another noteworthy point about this dream is that the psyche of the woman spoke in a symbolic language that could be understood by the homeopath. Once a healing alliance is made, the psyche often chooses language that the therapist can understand. Someone under Freudian analysis will have Freudian dreams. In Jungian analysis, the patient will have dreams that can be understood by a Jungian-trained analyst. The same principle can work with homeopathic patients. The adaptability of the psyche to communicate what the patient needs is a wonderful example of how, given a supportive environment, the psyche assists in the healing process, yet another way for the homeopath to understand the communication of the vital force.

The "Dreaming" Physician

The first step in creating a supportive environment in which to develop communication with the patient's psyche is by following one's own dreams. Practitioners who work with their dreams will become more familiar with the language of the psyche and with their own inner landscape.

Keeping a dream journal is an essential part of this process, as it gives a message to the "dream maker" that it will be heard. This process includes having the intention of remembering a dream and writing the dream in a journal on awakening. This will stimulate the dream state and help one remember dreams. All of the details immediately remembered from the dream are written in the journal and filled in with details that the writing process itself calls to mind. After this, comments and feelings about the dream are added without any consideration for logic and without editing the thoughts. The dream state is not logical or rational, and no attempt should be made to make it so.

Another helpful practice is to tell the dream to someone. Even if the listener cannot interpret the dream, the process of recounting the dream can stimulate insight into its meaning. If one does not have the good fortune of having a professional therapist who works with dreams, then a dream partner—a friend or acquaintance with whom to exchange dreams—can be of great assistance. It is said that Jung had trouble finding a professional who could understand his dreams, so he told his dreams to his gardener.

The Senoi people of Malaysia, whose society puts great emphasis on dream work, say that there are three parts to a dream. The first part is the experience of dreaming the dream. The second part is the telling of the dream, and the third part is the interpretation of the dream. Until all three parts are experienced, the dream is incomplete. The dream partner is especially important here because it is difficult to interpret one's own dreams. The dream is often telling us something that we are unwilling to see, though the meaning may be obvious to almost anyone else.

The technique of dream analysis will be discussed in depth in a later chapter, but the following example will give an idea of how to proceed in dream analysis with a dream partner.

Suppose you write a dream in a dream journal in the following way:

THURSDAY MORNING JANUARY 24, 2002

> *A white elephant is flying over the house where I lived with my mother and father. A young girl is standing outside with her bicycle looking up at the flying elephant.*
>
> *Your comments: The young girl seems in awe of the flying elephant. I wake up wondering what the dream means. The day before, I felt tired and was wondering when I would have my next vacation.*

The dreamer then tells the dream to the dream partner, who asks about all parts of the dream. What is this elephant? This one is white—why would you dream of a white elephant? Is it flying with wings, or just flying? How old is the little girl? What is your association to living in that house? What about the bicycle?

You go through all parts of the dream in this way in order to explore each symbol. Each can be seen as something outside of yourself, but much more frequently, the symbols of the dream relate to your inner state. The dream can be looked at in both ways. Finally, the dream partner will ask how the dream relates to what is going on in your life at the present time. A good sign that the dream is understood is the experience of an "Aha!" in which the message from the dream comes through and an issue suddenly becomes clear.

The above example, being theoretical, is very flat and uninspiring compared to the richness of a meaningful genuine dream. As continuing to work with dreams and the contents of the internal landscape become more familiar, the psyche will begin to communicate in increasingly complex and meaningful ways. These symbolic messages will act as guides and add to self-knowledge. Meeting one's more undesirable and hidden shadow side will most likely be an early experience in the journey to self-knowledge. If not daunted by the humbling process of seeing the dark side of the personality, you may be able to explore other archetypal realms that lie beneath the surface of the conscious mind.

Along with guiding the journey into self-discovery, the process of dream analysis is an essential step in building a bridge between the therapist and the patient's dreams. It is this bridge that both stand upon as they explore the symbols contained within the ocean of the unconscious.

Although this chapter has focused on the medical use of dreams and symbols, once a connection to this realm has been made, one also connects to the agenda of the psyche, which is rarely limited to the reduction of physical symptoms. Dreams and symbols point to a greater reality, to a truth about life that is yet unknown and by which one is drawn into the process of discovery and transformation. Jung addresses this point at the end of his chapter on the practical use of dream–analysis in *The Practice of Psychotherapy*. "The way of successive assimilations goes far beyond the curative results that specifically concern the doctor," he writes. "It leads in the end to that distant goal which may perhaps have been the first urge to life: the complete actualization of the whole human being, that is, individuation. We physicians may well be the first conscious observers of this dark process of nature. As a rule we see only the pathological phase of development, and we lose sight of the patient as soon as he is cured. Yet it is only after the cure that we would really be in a position to study the normal process, which may extend over years and decades."[6]

CHAPTER NINE

Case Taking

Perceiving What Needs to Be Healed

The purpose of the homeopathic interview is to perceive what needs to be healed in an individual and to gather enough information to divine the unique complex of characteristic signs and symptoms underlying the obvious and common symptoms of the patient's disease. The information leading to the correct remedy, or simillimum, is often hidden underneath massive amounts of a disease's common symptoms, side effects of medication, and ideas and attitudes that the patient has assimilated from others. In some patients, the key to the case will be found in symptoms that lie in the realm of consciousness, and in others, it is hidden in the unconscious.

The goal of dream analysis in case taking is to enrich symptoms that are reported by the patient and those observed by the homeopath with material from the symbolic realm of the unconscious. Dreams and symbols are connections to the ancient realm of the collective unconscious and must be linked with more conscious information in order to be useful. No dream or symbol has meaning outside the context of the whole person. Dreams are not shortcuts to understanding an individual; they are a rich and complex way to delve deeply into the underlying structures of the individual psyche as it is connected with the timeless region of the collective unconscious. Since one of the most common ways for the unconscious to communicate is through dreams and symbols, it is for homeopaths to have ears to hear and eyes to see the language of the dream state.

The intelligence of the psyche has access to more information and creativity than can be held by the individual consciously. The psyche knows with whom to communicate and in what way. So, only if the homeopath has the ability to understand will the patient's psyche bother to send messages through dreams that are relevant to the therapy. For this reason, it is important for homeopaths to develop a relationship to the dream state and their own psyches through dream journaling and sharing dreams with a partner.

The initial part of case taking with dreams is a process that one prepares for by developing receptivity toward and respect for the psyche. This receptive attitude coupled with active listening becomes an invitation, an opportunity, for the psyche of the patient to communicate with the homeopath. It opens up a stream of psychic flow between the psyche of the patient and the psyche of the homeopath that is the essence of the healing relationship.

Within this healing relationship, an individual will produce dreams that can be understood by the therapist. Homeopathic patients often tell dreams that point to the remedy they need. Even if the dream was dreamt years ago, it is one of thousands of dreams a patient has had in the past. The fact that a particular dream is remembered during the interview is of special significance. The dream often contains a clue to the remedy and is a tool the patient's vital force uses to point to meaning in what may appear to be chaos.

Although the timing will, of course, vary from situation to situation, it is preferable to ask about dreams after a complete case has been taken. In other words, after the person has given all of the information he or she is going to volunteer—including modalities, generals, and family history—then comes the time to ask about dreams. The homeopath might ask, "What dreams did you have in your childhood that you still remember today?" Or, "What dreams do you have that repeat over and over?" "What did you dream last night?" and "Tell me about the most significant dream you have ever had."

The information revealed in dream analysis is often a second story that is symbolic but parallel to the information in the initial case taking. After telling a dream, patients may begin to speak on another level, one that is much more personal and intimate. It is here that they may tell their deepest desires, especially if the dream is one that has been remembered from childhood. Frequently, the synchronicity between the dream and the contents of the rest of the case will be revealed at this time, and the revelation is often profound and delightful.

The Psychological Types

Another important factor that nurtures the possibility for communication on this deep and healing level is the rapport that is established between the homeopath and the patient. No homeopath, no matter how much they know and how in tune with their psyche, can be in rapport with all patients.

Jung divided people into different types according to their attitudes and ways in which they function. Though explaining the Jungian types in depth would fill many books,[1] it is worth mentioning here the relevance of Jungian typology to the homeopath. Although the typology of the patient is an important consideration, in the matter of case taking, homeopaths would do well to first understand the strengths and weaknesses of their own typology. A word of caution: While the psychological types are helpful in learning about people, they are not dogma but, rather, a practical way of looking at different styles of functioning. In addition, determining an individual type is not something that can be done quickly. Jung once quipped, not completely in humor, that often an individual's type can only be known when looking at his entire biography thirty years after his death. Understanding one's own type can be a challenge, but it is helpful to at least understand that people operate differently.

Extravert and Introvert

The two basic attitudinal types, according to Jung, are the extravert and the introvert, and they are defined by the flow of psychic energy: The extravert's psychic energy flows outward toward objects in the world, while the introvert's energy preference is an inward flow toward the subjective world. These attitudinal types are connected with the basic temperament or tendencies and can be seen even in the very young child. Although most people are not completely in one attitude or the other, everyone will have one attitude that is conscious and dominant, as well as an unconscious, opposite, and inferior attitude. As we shall later see, the inferior attitudes and functions, because they are not consciously utilized, remain in a more undeveloped state. This can be compared to the dominance in handedness. If the right hand is dominant, then the left hand is less developed and vice versa.

Extraverts relate directly to the world around them and receive energy from that contact. They are outgoing and like to make contact with others through either friendliness or argument. Highly suggestible and prone to the influence of other people, extraverts may express themselves through the ideas of others. The unconscious of extraverts must compensate for the continual focus on the external by becoming introverted. If extraverts focus so entirely on the outside world that they lose sight of their inner self and their body, the psyche creates physical symptoms that force the individual to turn inward. This is the typical neurosis of the extraverted type, and many extraverted people who have physical symptoms that do not respond to conventional treatment fall into this category.

Extraverted homeopaths are able to meet and connect with people easily. Because they gain energy from contacts with people and objects outside of themselves, they have good endurance and can bear the demands of a large practice. They can, however, become so involved in work that they forget to take care of themselves and can eventually become ill from overwork.

In contrast, introverts must constantly defend themselves from outside influences in order to conserve their energy and are more concerned with their feelings, impressions, and emotions. Their relationship to the outside world is centered on how it relates to their internal world, a state that can appear to be egocentric. The introverted state is, however, an inherited tendency present before ego development and therefore relates to all internal or psychic contents, not just to the ego alone. There is, however, a danger in introversion that, if the ego identifies with an archetypal configuration (for example, the archetype of the healer), it may become inflated with delusions of grandeur. The unconscious must then compensate by producing overwhelming fears that prevent action in the world and debilitate the individual with the enervation and anxiety typical of the neurotic state in the introvert.

The strengths of introverted homeopaths include sensitivity to the subjective states that are represented in the suffering of the patient and in the homeopathic remedies themselves. Because introverted homeopaths focus primarily on the internal realm of the psyche, these homeopaths inspire communication from that level in their patients. Dream analysis is a natural outcome of this type of interaction. These homeopaths are, however, prone to exhaustion and chronic fatigue when working with a large number of people and must be careful to replenish their energy with periods of the inner reflection from which they draw their psychic energy.

The Functional Types

According to Jung, there are four basic functions—thinking, feeling, intuition, and sensation—each of which can be either introverted or extraverted. He categorized two of the basic functions as rational and two as irrational. The thinking and feeling functions have to do with judging; weighing right and wrong, like and dislike. The sensation and intuitive functions are about perception. Jung called the judging types of thinking and feeling rational and the perception types of sensation and intuition irrational. I find those terms confusing and prefer to use the terms *judging* and *perception* for these two subcategories of the four functions. Knowledge of an individual's specific type is essential in Jungian analysis. What is more useful and perhaps more possible for homeopaths is to understand their own type, because each functional type will have a different style of case taking and analysis. This awareness also allows homeopaths to accept their own strengths and weakness and to improve the secondary functions. Knowledge of the Jungian functional types is of particular importance for teachers of homeopathy who, given this understanding, are better able to guide students into their own strengths in case taking.

Understanding one's own typology also creates a basis for understanding that patients will be of different types and have different ways of relating to the world. The many different categories of people who need the same remedy can be partially understood through the different types. An extraverted thinking type who needs *Sulfur,* for instance, will look very different from an introverted intuitive person needing *Sulfur.* The former may more closely resemble the outgoing, practical idealist and the latter the ragged philosopher type.

The Four Functions

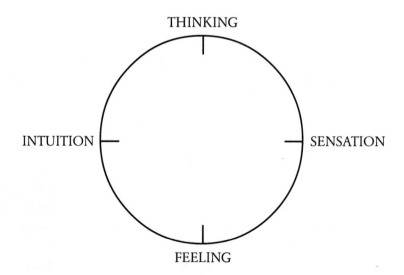

An important aspect of Jungian typology is the recognition that the inferior function is the individual's weakest function. Since people often develop more than one strong function, it may be difficult to tell which one is primary. Since the inferior function is always the opposite of the primary function, we can discern the primary function through a person's weakness and difficulty. For example, if a person has both strong intuition and strong thinking functions, it is difficult to see which is primary. However, if we find that they have great difficulty with feelings, are somewhat undifferentiated in that area and always getting into trouble with their feelings, they are most likely a thinking type. The feeling function is always inferior in the thinking type (see diagram).

Example of an Extraverted Thinking Type

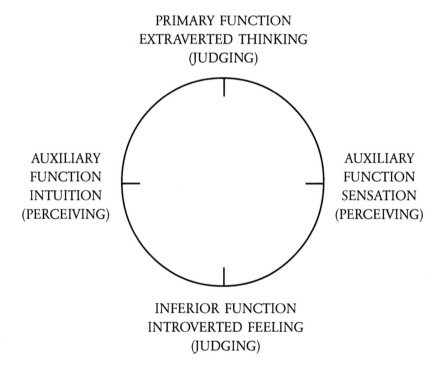

PRIMARY FUNCTION
EXTRAVERTED THINKING
(JUDGING)

AUXILIARY
FUNCTION
INTUITION
(PERCEIVING)

AUXILIARY
FUNCTION
SENSATION
(PERCEIVING)

INFERIOR FUNCTION
INTROVERTED FEELING
(JUDGING)

The inferior function is always the least developed of the four functions and the one that is very difficult for an individual to develop. However, the inferior function has a very important role: Being more primitive and less conscious, it serves as the door to the unconscious.

The Thinking Function

The thinking function drives the individual toward structure, order, and meaning. When most of a person's actions proceed from intellectually considered motives, that person is most likely a thinking type. Extraverted thinking is focused on an external object or person and is a deliberate act of rational judgment, whereas introverted thinking is more concerned with ideas and the logical process of the mind.

Homeopaths who are extraverted thinking types, for example, will develop a formula or a system within which to work. Their ability to organize and categorize the information in a case is very strong. They have a tendency try to fit the individual into a preconceived idea that is part of their intellectual formula: This is the inherent danger when one organizes information within a system and then falls in love with the system. Extraverted thinking homeopath's can also have difficulty with the feeling function that is the least developed or inferior function. The feelings of this type tend to be undeveloped and undifferentiated, and these people may appear cold or react negatively to someone who challenges their system. In working with dreams, these homeopaths will be tempted to work with dream books that present formulas for symbols and to develop systems categorizing dreams belonging to different remedy types. This type of categorization, although interesting, is not truly helpful in working with dreams, as it is the dreamer's associations to the dream that are of primary importance. With the possible exception of the relative similarity found in archetypal symbols, each dream is unique to the dreamer and is affected by the psyche of the homeopath to whom it is told.

Introverted thinking type homeopaths are more concerned with ideas and the way that the mind organizes itself. They generally have a good ability to wait and see how the information in a case evolves into a pattern rather than attempting to fit it into a formula. They have the ability to organize information in a case, but because extraverted feeling is the inferior function, they may have difficulty with feelings that come about during the interview. These homeopaths may also have trouble with emotional boundaries and must take care not to step over them. Dreams are interesting to these types because dreams gives the homeopaths access to the organization of the psyche, something that is of great interest to them. Because of the introverted thinking types' ability to ascertain order and meaning, they are able to utilize the information from the dream in relation to the rest of the case. They should be aware, however not to ignore the feelings expressed in the dreams.

The Feeling Function

The feeling function makes a judgment about internal or external objects based on likes and dislikes. In its normal state, the judgment is calm and can be very accurate; only if the feeling crosses into emotion is it no longer a "rational" feeling. Extraverted feeling is focused on the individual's environment, and his or her relation to the environment takes on great importance. Introverted feeling is more hidden and influences the environment indirectly.

Homeopaths who are of the extraverted feeling type have the ability to connect with people and have few illusions about them. People speak to them openly, because extraverted feeling types have an air of acceptance and friendliness, a valuable asset in a homeopath. However, this type's intense desire to stay in rapport with everyone may prevent him or her from asking awkward but sometimes necessary questions in the interview. Their desire to stay in rapport with the patient may make dealing with irritations and healing crises difficult for them.

The extraverted feeling type's inferior function, which is introverted thinking, may create a challenge for these types, because they dislike thinking, as it interferes with their feeling process. What they cannot feel they cannot consciously think. This may stand in the way of their ability to guide the patient into giving the right information while taking the case and prevent objective case analysis.

Dream work is interesting to these homeopaths, because of the feeling expressed in many dreams. However, if dreams are violent or contain many mixed emotions, these homeopaths can become confused. It is a challenge for them to leave the world of the emotions and help patients analyze their dreams by looking at the structure or a specific part of the dream. To the feeling type, such a procedure might seem more like an autopsy than an analysis.

The introverted feeling types are a difficult type to understand. They tend to exert a positive influence on society while remaining in the background. Homeopaths who have introverted feeling as their primary function may have difficulty relating to patients because the type assumes indifference as a means of defense and tends to shrink away from any the outward expression of strong emotion. Their inferior function, extraverted thinking, causes them to get lost in a morass of details, as they are people who focus on one or very few ideas. This would make case analysis difficult unless they always approached a case in the same way. For example, if the introverted feeling type were interested in dream analysis, he or she might adopt Freud's idea of relating all symbols to one source. Jung once said that Freudian psychology was typical of the inferior extraverted thinking function because it was based on very few repetitive ideas.

The Intuitive Function

The function of intuition is unconscious perception. An idea emerges whole and complete without the person's being able to explain how it developed. Because of this, intuitive types have the ability to see many possibilities without being inhibited by logic. They see the big picture and can often predict events before they happen. Extraverted intuitive types have perceptions about the outside world, while introverted intuitive types perceive inner psychic data.

Extraverted intuitive-type homeopaths have wonderful imaginations and can see many possibilities in a case. Often rightly accused of being vague, these types cannot, when challenged, put their finger on how they actually came up with a remedy. They are fond of using many different types of case analysis, becoming bored with doing just one thing. This restlessness can lead them to change professions after practicing for a while. Their inferior function, introverted sensation, makes it difficult for them to see all of the details in a case, and they may tire of the slowness of precise case taking. The novelty and newness of each dream will appeal to these homeopaths, and they will often sense the many levels of meaning in a dream. However, since these homeopaths prefer to look at things vaguely in order to stimulate their intuition, they may not have the patience to look at the different parts of the dream with the patient.

Homeopaths of the introverted intuitive type will be able to "pull the remedy out of the hat" by leaps of intuition, as they play with the archetypes of remedies within the psyche. Vagueness about facts, however, is their downfall. The inferior function, extraverted sensation, makes it difficult for them to see the details and concrete symptoms in the case.

Dreams are home to introverted intuitive homeopaths, who live among the subjective dimensions of the psyche. Often, the meaning of the dream comes to them in the typical intuitive flash. The challenge for introverted intuitive homeopaths is to ground their intuition in the details of the dream and to allow the patient to make the associations, and to resist the urge to impose their intuitive flash on the analysis.

The Sensation Function

The function of sensation is conscious perception and is identical to sense perception. The senses are alert and pick up differences in texture, sounds, odors, and colors. When extraverted sensation types walk into a room, they take a picture of everything going on. These types notice the people in the room and what they are wearing and would make great spies, because they notice any little difference in detail. Introverted sensation types have the same sensing abilities but the information from the outside makes an impression deep inside of them. Often, they can express these impressions through writing or painting.

Homeopaths who are sensation types, whether extraverted or introverted, are excellent gatherers of information. They miss very little in a case and notice all of the details, an excellent skill for a homeopath. When practitioners take three hours or so to take a case, it is very likely that they are sensation types. Their inferior function, intuition, may contribute not only to a lack of imagination, but can also cause them to distain and suspect anything approaching that realm. These types have a tendency to dismiss new and imaginative ideas as quackery and ineptness.

Working with dreams is more mechanical for sensation types, who can easily go through all the parts of the dream with the dreamer. It is sometimes difficult for them to make the leap into how the information from the dream fits into the rest of the case and how it relates to a remedy.

Homeopaths who are introverted sensation types are similar to the extraverted type, except that the impressions that are made on them affect them deeply. This tends to delay their reactions, so these types may have to let the case "brew" for several days before the information registers. Their inferior function, extraverted intuition, can haunt these people through prophetic fantasies, as the undeveloped intuition has a weird and eerie quality for them.

The details required in dream analysis come easily to introverted sensation types, and they will slowly move through the dream with the patient. Because they need time to register what is going on, they may have trouble guiding the patient during the analysis.

Judgment and Perception

Many people have a secondary function that is fairly well developed. In homeopaths, such a development is essential because the secondary function creates the ability to use both judgment and perception in case taking. In other words, if the primary function is a judging function, either thinking or feeling, the secondary function will be a perceiving function, either intuition or sensation.

Because judgment is concerned with evaluation, the homeopath assessing the patient through judgment will see the more conscious, concrete aspect of the individual. The homeopath will consciously use his or her ability to discriminate between the pieces of information that the patient conveys. Conversely, the homeopath working from perception will be in touch with the more unconscious character because perception reveals the individual's process, the underlying flow beneath the bits of information represented by symbols, and other subtle information not as easily available to judgment. Given this, the homeopath must be able to use both judgment and perception while conducting the initial interview, for it is possible for the guiding symptoms that lead to the correct remedy to lie within the more conscious, concrete symptoms or within a symbolic representation of the unconscious state. Furthermore, the pattern of guiding symptoms often weaves in and out between the conscious and unconscious state, making it impossible for the homeopath to perceive what needs to be healed unless he or she is able to use both perception and judgment in case taking.

In order for the intuitive logic of the symbolic realm to reveal itself, the therapist must be able to discriminate between the information that fits into the pattern that repeats itself within the information presented by the patient and information that is extraneous. Working within the symbolic realm requires that the therapist remain open to seeing this repetitive pattern without coming to a premature conclusion as to its nature. To do this requires the simultaneous use of both perception and judgment. To jump to conclusions and make a premature judgment is to overlay another reality, generated by the intellect, upon the emerging pattern. One must be willing to suspend judgment and be in a state of not knowing while simultaneously discriminating between what may be useful and what is not.

This vacillation between the judging operation of the intellect and the more receptive aspect of perception eventually reveals an entirely new and holistic understanding of the case, a holographic picture not unlike the imagery created in dreams.

Therapists can cultivate the ability to maintain the state of "not knowing" and prepare themselves to be receptive toward the dreams and symbolic language of their patients by working with their own dreams and practicing some form of meditation.

Even a rudimentary understanding of the psychological types can give homeopaths an understanding that there is a basic difference in the way that individuals perceive and report their symptoms. This understanding helps the homeopath avoid the mistake of being thrown off balance by the patient's particular style of functioning. Being aware of their own function also helps homeopaths avoid projecting their style of functioning onto the patient, a phenomenon known as projection or transference.

Transference

Transference is the projection of one's psychic contents onto another person or object, one's shadow material being a favorite. Projection is something that happens in all encounters, and more often when the inner state has not been examined. I experienced a vivid example of this a few years ago while on a weeklong silent retreat for *vipassana* meditation.

A friend and I attended a retreat where, along with about a hundred other people, we were to remain in silence and be mindful of what was going on in our inner state. We all meditated and ate together without interacting through words or eye contact. On the long drive home after spending the week in silence, my friend and I entertained one another with the way we had projected our inner feelings and thoughts on our unassuming retreat partners. We could not stop laughing at the ridiculousness of the stories we had made up about other people. Hardly any of this was based in reality; it was all a projection of our inner state onto the people around us. This phenomenon is so common that vipassana teachers often talk of the imaginary relationships that people have during retreat. During the week of silence, one can, in one's own mind, fall in love, get married, and finally divorce someone without even speaking to him or her.

This phenomenon of transference goes on all the time and in all relationships. The only difference between the meditation course and everyday life is that we were being mindful, so we saw it happening. This mindfulness or awareness is a first step in realizing how much of what is thought to be reality is a manifestation of our own projection.

In therapy, *transference* refers to the patient projecting the contents of their psyche onto the therapist, and *countertransference* refers to the therapist's projection, the process in reverse. Freud warned that therapists needed to protect themselves from transference. While he was aware of the dangers, Jung considered transference as inevitable and part of the healing alliance.

"The transference itself is a perfectly natural phenomenon which does not by any means happen only in the consulting room," Jung wrote in *The Practice of Psychotherapy*. "It can be seen everywhere and may lead to all sorts of nonsense, like all unrecognized projections. Medical treatment of the transference gives the patient a priceless opportunity to withdraw his projections, to make good his losses, and to integrate his personality."[2]

Homeopaths are not immune to the phenomenon of transference and countertransference just because it is not generally acknowledged in the field. In fact, the most dangerous aspect of transference is not being aware that it exists. A continual and unconscious exposure to the projections of patients can leave homeopaths in the situation of unconsciously developing a persona. Adopting this persona is like putting on a mask or a second skin for the purpose of protection and can be a state of outward irritability, coldness, or phony niceness by which one can become possessed. An old movie, *Morgan,* demonstrates this phenomenon. In it, a young man is fascinated by gorillas and often dresses in a gorilla suit. The gorilla suit can be compared to the persona, a mask that we wear to protect ourselves. The persona is only a problem when we are not conscious of what we are doing. When we unconsciously develop a persona, we begin to identify with it. We begin to think that the persona is who we are. At the end of the movie, Morgan puts on the gorilla suit and can't remove it; he has become completely identified with it. Homeopaths would do well to check in the mirror for unwanted fur.

Awareness of the phenomenon of transference is a most important first step in dealing with it. In the initial homeopathic interview, homeopaths must be able to separate their projections from the reality of the patient's state. Otherwise, an entirely false picture of the person can be made up based on the projection. If the patient touches or resonates with one's own psychological state, this becomes more of a problem. Knowing oneself is a vital step in achieving a clearer perception of another.

In order to separate out their personal emotions from the emotions of the patient, homeopaths can monitor their dreams for clues. If a patient keeps appearing in a dream, it may mean that the homeopath has taken in some of that person's psychic state. Supervision of your psychic state by another homeopath or a therapist is also helpful. If there is too much transference or countertransference the patient may need to be referred to another practitioner because it can become impossible to see the case clearly, creating a situation injurious to both the homeopath and the patient.

Although psychotherapy uses the word *countertransference* to indicate the projections of therapists and its effects on them, the reality of the situation is that the healing alliance profoundly affects both the homeopath and the patient. The deeper the problem and the longer the patient and homeopath work together, the more important the quality of this alliance. Ideally, the transference allows the homeopath to become the crucible, the alchemical vessel that holds the essence of the patient in the process of transformation.

The Crucible

All that is visible must grow beyond itself, extend into the realm of the invisible. Thereby it receives its true consecration and clarity and takes firm root in the cosmic order.

THE I CHING[3]

Information that is received during case taking, including dream material, is the undistilled substance in need of alchemical transformation—what the alchemists called the *prima materia*. The transformation of this material into an essence that will finally lead to the simillimum is similar to the alchemical process of *separatio*, in which the alchemist separates the parts of a substance in order put them back together in a way that transforms the whole. Once homeopaths have investigated and "potentized" a certain amount of their own psychic contents through making them conscious, homeopaths may act as an alchemical vessel, or crucible, that separates the characteristic symptoms from the plethora of information offered. These symptoms must then go through a second transformation, that of coniunctio, or conjunction (used in alchemy to refer to chemical combinations), in which the parts are reassembled in a way that reveals the *"Imbegriff der symptome,"* a phrase used by Hahnemann to indicate the totality of characteristic symptoms in a case, which may also be translated as the essence or quintessence of the case. Because homeopaths serve as crucibles in which the essence of the case is temporarily contained and transformed, they have one more reason to understand the dynamics of their own psyches. The more homeopaths are imprisoned by their complexes, the more these unconscious complexes filter the stream of information coming from the client. The more aware the homeopaths are of their own psychic terrain, the less that terrain will interfere and the more knowledge and energy will be liberated for the patient's benefit. In *The Alchemy of Healing*, Edward Whitmont describes how therapists' awareness of complexes can benefit the healing process:

> *Inevitably complexes corresponding or similar to those of the patient are activated in the healer ... when the healer unconsciously acts out those complexes, they operate like poison and add to the patient's disturbance. Conversely, when "potentized" into symbolic awareness by the healer, they help the healing process.*[4]

This crucible is not only an arena for the separating out of the essence from the *prima materia* of a case; the crucible also functions as a holding place for the transference during the healing process. This means that the homeopath is always in danger of taking on some of the suffering of the client. This sacrifice is part of the work.

Fortunately the remedy also holds some aspect of the transference. Moreover, unlike psychotherapists, homeopaths share the burden of the transference with the remedy. Nevertheless, because it is very tempting for the homeopath to take credit for the whole process, that is, to identify with what is held within the collective unconscious as well as the healing effect of the remedy, the most dangerous pitfall is inflation. In inflation, the ego identifies with the entire healing process and thus falls prey to grandiosity and delusions of power. Adolf Guggenbühl-Craig, a Swiss Jungian psychoanalyst, addresses this problem in *Power in the Helping Professions:*

> *At the start of therapy, the relation between the therapist and patient is often like that of the sorcerer and his apprentice. And the patient's sorcerer-and-apprentice fantasies have a very powerful effect on the therapist, in whose unconscious the figure of the magician or savior begins to be constellated. The therapist starts to think that he is in fact someone with supernatural powers, capable of working wonders with his magic.*[5]

Later in his book, Guggenbühl-Craig makes a case for how difficult it is for someone in the helping profession to get help with inflation. Patients only make it worse by transferring their expectations onto therapists, and others in the profession have too much to lose to exclaim that the emperor has no clothes. Guggenbühl-Craig feels that help lies in having good and trustworthy friends who will let you know when you are getting out of line. Homeopaths may also benefit from having a partner or supervisor to whom they can tell their dreams, because dreams will often send messages that compensate inflation.

Incorporating dream analysis into the initial homeopathic interview requires that homeopaths prepare themselves to be receptive to the psyche by developing respect for and becoming familiar with its symbolic language.

Whether this symbolism appears in dreams, in the actual language of the patient, or is found in the characteristic symptoms of the physical disease, it may serve as a guiding symptom when used along with other characteristic symptoms. Understanding the psychic processes, such as projection, and the different types of functions is important in sifting out extraneous information that may stand in the way of clearly perceiving what needs to be healed.

Ultimately the homeopathic interview is a unique experience in which one human being enters into a completely new realm with another in order to discover a pattern that connects a being to a substance in the form of a homeopathic remedy. Given the number of physical substances in the universe and the intricacy of the body/mind, it is a small miracle that a matching pattern can be found at all. The simillimum is only found because there is an inherent order and wisdom that is constantly pointing the way through the symptoms generated by the vital force of the individual. It is only necessary to step out of the way and follow that lead.

CHAPTER TEN

Communicating with the Psyche
The Subtle Technique of Dream Analysis

Dream analysis is less about knowing and more about not knowing. It is best done with what the Zen teacher Shunryu Suzuki has called "beginner's mind."[1] "In the beginner's mind," he writes, "there are many possibilities, but in the expert's there are few." Dream analysis is most fruitful when one is open to many possibilities by admitting ignorance. Drawing premature conclusions about the meaning of a dream is the biggest danger.

The role of dream analysis in homeopathic treatment may be different than in psychoanalysis, but the technique is the same. Jung's aim in dream analysis was to become aware of previously unreachable contents of the psyche, the knowledge of which was important in the treatment of a neurosis. The aim in homeopathic treatment is to use the dream to help elucidate the repeating pattern in a person's history and vital force that will shed light both on what needs to be cured in the individual and on the remedy that will cure it through the law of similars. Some homeopaths call this repeating pattern the "red thread" that runs through a case. Dreams allow the psyche to reveal the unconscious background of the conscious state, so that what was once hidden can be used to help find the correct remedy and further the healing process.

In a successful analysis, the dreamer contemplates the dream, and the therapist guides the dreamer into communication with his own psyche. When this process is successful, the dreamer can often retrieve "buried treasure"—golden nuggets that are essential to both parties' understanding of what needs to be healed.

Because the main idea is to receive the message from the unconscious, the therapist must not assume to know anything, nor suggest any meaning.

Jung called treatments based on suggestion "deceptive makeshifts" that are incompatible with the principles of analytic therapy. In homeopathic terms, suggestions are either palliative or suppressive actions that, although sometimes helpful in particular circumstances, are not part of the curative process.

One must be careful not to reduce the symbolic imagery to narrow easy answers like "a cow jumping over the moon means problems with a hysterical mother." These kinds of dream interpretations are often found in unsophisticated books on dream analysis and are better off being disregarded. Even well-educated opinions about a dream are chancy, as one can never be sure of being right. It is better to rely on the associations of the dreamer and the actual facts of the dream for the interpretation.

The homeopath can think of the dream as a map of the psyche, which is a real place, just like the body, where the different parts—the arms, the liver, and so forth—relate to the whole. Dreams are facts about the psychic state, about needs and difficulties that can only be understood in relation to an individual's entire life. One must know the person before even beginning to understand the dream. Even within the context of the whole person, the dream can never be totally understood. It shows the unconscious aspect of an event in the form of symbolic imagery generated by the psyche, and the psyche cannot know its own psychic substance. Said in another way, we cannot totally understand the human mind, because it must be studied by the mind.

Each dream is a unique expression. Although there are some helpful guidelines and techniques that assist in revealing the messages generated by dreams, each encounter is a new experience. In each case, one must to be able to give up all theories and preconceived ideas and return to "beginner's mind."

Free Association and Dream Analysis

Sigmund Freud was the first to attempt to understand the unconscious in relationship to consciousness in an empirical way. His exploration led him to use dreams and to elucidate them through a process of free association. He allowed his patients to talk about their dream images in order to reveal the unconscious contents of their minds and to help him understand their neuroses. Although free association is helpful in leading an individual to deeper levels of the psyche, it is not specific to the symbolism generated by the actual dream. Jung discovered that one could free associate on almost anything, and the free association would lead to the basic underlying complexes within the psyche.

The dream, according to Jung, generates some very specific symbolic imagery, and it is this imagery that must be explored. When we explore the specific content of dreams, we get much more precise information. The dreamer is never allowed to move too far away from the dream's symbols and themes. He or she must concentrate on the specifics of the dream, because resistance to ideas that may create a change or conflict within the individual and fear of new and unknown ideas emerging from the dream imagery often lead the dreamer away from these contents into the realm of free association. When this happens, it is essential to bring the dreamer back to the specifics of the dream.

Not only the dreamer, however, can become frustrated and move away from the contents of the dream. At times, the interpreter can become stymied by the difficulty of understanding certain symbolism and will be tempted to either dismiss the dream or to "theorize" about its meaning. If the dream is to be understood at all, both dreamer and interpreter must stay as close to the specifics as possible.

Levels of Dream Analysis

Dreams can be understood on many levels, which can be divided into three categories: the literal, the psychological, and true communication with the unconscious. The literal is the rational approach, which uses the intellect to understand the symbolic imagery and reduces it to what is known about the symbol. In this way, the symbols of the dream are restricted and are no longer used as symbols but rather as signs given a particular meaning by the intellect. This is the level of dream analysis addressed by many so-called dream books. This level of dream analysis is not at all helpful in determining what needs to be cured in the individual and should not be used by the homeopath.

The second, or psychological, level of dream analysis is more sophisticated but not as useful when it comes to understanding the symbolic content of a dream. Here the attempt is to relate the dreams to the psychological situation of the dreamer. This is the way that many psychotherapists work with dreams. It is the realm of psychotherapy and should not be practiced by anyone without training in that profession. The psychological meaning of the dream is much less useful in the practice of homeopathy than the third level of analysis.

The third level of analysis comes from the unconscious, and in order for the dreamer to understand a dream on this level, the dreamer must be open to his or her unconscious. It is much more important that the interpretation feels right to the dreamer than to the therapist. Often, various interpretations must be tried until one fits; then it is as if a bell goes off and both the dreamer and therapist understand a whole new truth signaled by the dream. It is this interpretation that is most useful in determining what the psyche is attempting to communicate. The facts of the dream then lead to an understanding that may be a significant symptom in finding the correct remedy.

For instance, a woman with a history of early childhood abuse has a low white blood cell count and severe weakness but very few characteristic symptoms to point to the appropriate remedy. She has been undergoing homeopathic treatment for a while with good results, but her remedy has stopped working. She has the following dream.

> *I'm on some strange, hard, cold planet. My son and I were going to be killed. The aliens shape-shifted into gas that would kill us. I kept saying, "Life is eternal."*
>
> *We get into a pod and go to another planet. It's scary, but I know it's going to be OK. Men run out—I'm afraid now we'll die. We've come so far and now we are going to die. But we start trading things and everything is OK.*

In order for the dream to be useful, the actual contents must first be understood. She associates the gas with breathing in poison gas, dying, and popping out on the other side. It is the trading that saves her life in the dream. She associates the trading with the capacity for real communication—the ability to give and receive. More information is needed about this. Rather than theorizing about the trading, the homeopath asks her to say more about what it means to her. She says that what she needs to do this is to have more "belly consciousness," which she explains as being more connected with the physical world.

The dream is very specific. It says that, in order to save her life, she needs to be more connected with the physical world. This indicates the need for a remedy that will ground her. Now the parts of the dream start to fall into place. The bell has gone off. Going to another planet is another way of expressing a lack of grounding—in the dream she is literally, not quite on this Earth. She has had to leave the strange hard, cold planet in order to survive.

The mechanism for her survival is a vehicle that brings her to another place where she can become more grounded and survive. It is important to use her specific words—she does not say *spaceship*. She refers to it as a pod. The dream speaks very specifically to the homeopath and indicates that the patient needs a remedy that will ground her and that the remedy is somehow associated with a pod.

Quite a few remedies will help ground a person, but only one is made from the pod of a plant and is known to help in cases where there is disassociation after post-traumatic stress disorder. That remedy is *Opium*, a remedy made from the pod of the opium poppy. After taking this remedy, the patient's energy improved. She felt more grounded, began exercising, and her white blood count returned to normal.

Subjective versus Objective Dreams

Dreams are often populated with people we know and events from daily life. This frequently leads to the theory that dreams are a mechanism by which the mind cleanses itself of the events of the day. Dreams about particular events and specific people, known as subjective dreams, are actually much more rare than dreams having to do with internal dynamics. Objective dreams are about the internal dynamics of the dreamer. The familiar people and places are actually symbolic representations of parts of the dreamer's psyche.

Although it can be difficult to discern if a dream is subjective or objective, looking at it both ways will usually point the way to the most useful interpretation. Inquiry into what happened in the dreamer's life previous to the dream may shed some light onto the matter. When people first begin to analyze their dreams, they tend to look at them subjectively. After a subjective analysis, the interpreter can suggest that the dreamer look at the dream as if all of the contents were part of the dreamer's internal state. This will give the dreamer a different and perhaps more enlightening perspective.

Steps of Dream Analysis

Although the process of dream analysis is highly individual, some steps can be taken to ensure the best possible results.

Listen to the entire dream and write down all parts of the dream. Avoid eliminating details that may seem unimportant.

After the dreamer has finished telling the dream and the interpreter has written it down, the dreamer should be allowed to tell his or her impression of it. If the dreamer begins to move away from the content of the dream, go back to the details by asking about the dream's specific contents.

Go through the entire dream in minute detail, asking for associations to all the images in the dream. Be specific, stay as close to the actual images as possible, and keep returning to the images. Many times, with dreamers who are just beginning to analyze their dreams, no associations will come to mind. If this happens, ask for more concrete associations to the image. For instance, if the dreamer has dreamed of a pig, ask the dreamer to describe it. The idea is to get the dreamer talking about his or her associations to pigs. Do this for all of the images—the objects, characters, and places—in the dream. If the dreamer moves away from the dream, keep steering back, returning to the image and staying rooted in the facts.

Once all of the dream images have been thoroughly explored, or at least described in detail, ask what conscious attitude the dream compensates for. In other words, a dream about having many relationships may be compensating for the fact that an individual is too insular and needs to have more contact with others. Without knowledge of the dreamer's everyday life, it is difficult to interpret the dream.

One can also ask about the general feeling or ambience of the dream and how that relates to the dreamer's current state. The ambience of a dream is often powerfully felt by both the dreamer and the therapist and is an essential part of dream analysis. Because this ambience is rarely transferred to the written word, it is often difficult to tell by reading about a dream how a therapist came to a particular conclusion regarding the dream's meaning.

After going through the details of the dream, comparing it to the dreamer's conscious attitude, and asking about the general feeling the dream conveys, the homeopath may be able to use the dream symbolism in the selection of the remedy. Although a particular symbol may relate directly to a remedy, more often it is the gestalt created by the dream meaning, along with the dream's ambience and relationship to the facts of a person's life, that is important. This gestalt, along with the rest of the characteristic symptoms of the case, is a reliable indicator of the remedy.

If the meaning of the dream is not clear, the homeopath should not settle for an easier explanation, as this will narrow the possibilities. Some dreams cannot be understood until much later. Other times, a dream is understood by the therapist, who must then hold this information for a while before the dreamer can understand it. This is one reason to keep a record of all of the dreams, with dates. If the patient is not capable of doing this, the homeopath must keep the record.

Other dreams are only understood in relationship to a series. When we hear a series of dreams, we can often be more certain about what is going on. In the bigger picture, an individual's dreams are a continuum, and if we could gather many of them over the length of a person's life, we might have a unique "road map" to the individual's psychic life.

If the homeopath and the client together arrive at a wrong conclusion about the meaning of a dream, the unconscious may react in the next dream so the interpretation can be corrected. The individual may have a dream, or a series of dreams, that points out the mistake and indicates the correct interpretation. When this happens, it can be something of an unwanted but useful gift to the therapist who will then have to then swallow his or her pride and admit to the misinterpretation. This "gift" will help the therapist who, due to the therapist's profession, is frequently in danger of self-inflation. The corrective dream will also be of use to the patient, who will now be less inclined to hold the therapist in a godlike role.

Archetypal Symbolism

Even though the personal association of the dreamer to the symbolism within the dream is of utmost importance, archetypal symbols in dreams will often have meaning that is more universal and larger than the individual. These symbols have ancient roots that move deep into the collective unconscious and are understood through their association with myths and motifs from many times and places. These symbols therefore require further research into their meaning, if the dream is to be understood. This research into myth, stories, and motifs will reveal many themes associated with the symbol that can then be applied to the more individual meaning that the symbol has for the dreamer. The realm of the archetype is, however, dangerous territory, because it is easy to become fascinated by the archetypal significance of the symbol and lose sight of the specifics of the dream itself. Therefore, bringing a larger perspective to bear on an individual's dream becomes a fine art that requires great discrimination.

The following dream, of a woman who has been undergoing Jungian analysis for many years, is an example how archetypal symbolism can relate to both the universal and the individual.

I'm sitting by a lake admiring swans. First there are white swans,
then gray swans. I'm reading a book about them: It says that the gray
swans appear in the spring. The gray swans are smaller, more graceful,
but I prefer the white ones.

The Penguin Dictionary of Symbols[2] refers to the symbolism of the swan as
representing the living manifestation of light in many cultures, both Eastern and Western. Traditionally, the swan can represent two different types
of light—the solar, male light of the sun and the female, lunar light of
night. The black swan represents the occult or more negative and lunar side
of the light, and white animals are often indicative of spirit. The ancient
alchemists associated the swan with Mercury, who was an expression of the
marriage of fire and water, the marriage of opposites.

This dream shows gray swans. Gray, the blending of both white and
black, relates to the marriage of opposites. So, we may think that this dream
has something to do with integration of the opposites in the dreamer's
psyche. She also says in the dream that, even though the gray swans are
more graceful, she prefers the white ones, indicating that she prefers to stay
on the white or spiritual side of things, away from the dark side.

But what about her personal associations to swans in general? She associates the swan with the story of the "Ugly Duckling." This is a story by Hans
Christian Andersen about a baby swan who grows up with ducks. Looking
quite different from all the cute, fuzzy, yellow ducklings, the swan feels ugly
because he is different and is ostracized and rejected by all of the animals
on the farm. The woman associates this story to her younger years, when
she was different from others and felt unappreciated. She suffered greatly
because of this and constantly felt misunderstood. After exploring the story,
she feels that the dream is telling her that, even though she felt out of place
and unsure of who she was in her younger years, she is moving into her
own unique self.

If we consider both the archetypal and the individual aspects of the
dream, we see that the imagery is telling a story of development—that which
has already taken place and that which is to come. As in the story the "Ugly
Duckling," the dreamer has developed into her own self, outside of her
family influence. But she still has an idealized view of who she is, prefer-
ring to be the more spiritual white swan rather than integrating the dark
and the light (the gray swans). The dream contains a hint, however, that this
development is to come, for in the dream, she reads a book that says the
gray swans appear in the spring.

This dream helped the patient understand that even though she had already integrated much of the dark side of her personality, she still was leaning too far toward the light or spiritual side. The dream also suggests that there will be a time (spring) when this integration will appear, indicating a process of healing pregnant with possibilities.

In a case like this, where we have symbolism that has deep archetypal significance, the more universal aspect of the symbol must be blended with the personal association in order to understand the dream. Usually, dreams that are useful in homeopathic practice are a blending of the archetypal and individual meaning. If, after receiving a remedy, a client has a dream such as the one about the swans, it would indicate to the homeopath that the remedy was working very deeply, because it predicts the possibility of greater integration.

The Trickster

Although dreams play no fixed role, their most frequent role is to compensate for the conscious state. In other words, a person who is very timid and has low self-confidence may have dreams of greatness. On the other hand, someone with an overdeveloped ego may dream of being a ragged beggar. All of this sounds very fine and logical, but in practice these dreams can be difficult to stomach, for they often play the role of the trickster, tricking or shaming one into greater balance.

Just as the trickster dispenses with polite formalities, the dream will often come right out and say what is going on. If the emperor has no clothes, the trickster has no difficulty in presenting naked imagery. Jung tells a story of a very opinionated woman known for her stubborn arguments. Her therapist tried to politely inform her of this with no effect. Then she had the following dream:

> *There is a great social affair to which she is invited. She is received by her hostess (a very bright woman) at the door with the words: "Oh, how nice that you have come, all your friends are already here and are expecting you." She leads her to a door, opens it, and the lady steps into a cow shed.*[3]

The woman didn't at first admit to the meaning of the dream, but she eventually accepted the self-inflicted joke.

When a dreamer is confronted with such a dream, it is useful to remind the person who has dreamed it. This prevents the patient from blaming the therapist for the imagery in order to escape from the healing sting of the message.

There is nothing that is sacred and cannot be grist for the trickster's mill. The psyche may create dream imagery that mirrors a negative quality in the therapist—and it can be in full color—as in the case of a woman who dreamed of her therapist as a fat, sloppy man smoking a cigar. The therapist was then the one who had to slink home with the image and think about what it was saying about him.

Once therapists begin to work with dreams, they are not immune to the process that the psyche has in store, and the therapist is no more protected from the slings and arrows of this process than is the patient. This danger, along with the irrational nature of dreams, is one of the reasons that many are hesitant to work with dreams. What is more useful than fearing what dreams may reveal is to develop a sense of humor.

The Initial Dreams

Certain dreams, known as initial dreams, will appear after a positive response to either the remedy or the healing alliance with the homeopath. They may also be dreams that are dreamt the night before the consultation. These dreams are often very clear and lucid and may possibly indicate the future outcome of the therapy, giving the homeopath an idea of what is ahead for the patient. An initial dream often brings forth a previously hidden or misunderstood origin.

Even though initial dreams may be lucid and clear, as work continues the dreams can appear to lose clarity. In actuality, the dreams are just as clear as ever, but sometimes the homeopath cannot follow them into the depth of the psychic process. It is important to admit to a lack of understanding when this happens. The homeopath must learn to tolerate the insecurity of not knowing, because working with dreams, as well as following the healing process, must, of necessity, lead into the realm of the unknown. On the other hand, the patient would like the homeopath to understand not only the dreams but also exactly where in the healing process the patient is. In actuality, nothing is worse than the therapist who always understands the patient, for this develops dependence. It is for the dreamer to connect with and become conscious of his or her own individual psychic process. It makes very little difference if the therapist understands the dream, but it makes all the difference if the patient understands.

Considerations in Dream Analysis

Two important factors to bear in mind when working with dreams are the dreamer's age and position in life. In the early part of life, up until about the age of forty, life should be more ego-centered and focused on the events of life, such as raising a family or developing a career. Dreams of younger people will be more concerned with outward concerns and ego development. If a young person is encouraged to focus on symbolism and the archetypes of the collective unconscious, the person may live in that realm instead of in the world, where they properly belong at this stage.

After midlife, a new focus develops, one that goes beyond the ego. This entails shifting from concerns about who one is and what one does in the world to an entirely new realm. If personal development is to continue, the separate identity, the building of which was the challenge of earlier life, must now be broken down to make way for a more expansive perspective. The ego must relinquish itself to a greater source; one that reaches beyond the personal or individual and into what Jung called the Self. This process requires development of another side of the personality in order to create wholeness. In the first part of life, certain abilities are developed based on personal strengths; later on the challenge is to develop other abilities that may have been neglected during the necessary ego-building period.

Most people past midlife tend to be very strongly rooted in their position in life. If they are imprisoned by their environment, the fantasy and symbolism of dreams can add great vitality and creativity to their lives. People of this age who have not developed their position in life, who are rootless, have entirely different goals. The imagery may serve as a way for them to escape into even more flights of fantasy. For some, the symbolic realm is the elixir of life; for others, the symbolic is an opiate that may keep these people from the challenges of their development.

It is helpful for the homeopath to understand these differences, especially in following the process of cure. Given the caveat that every individual is different, if, after the administration of a new remedy, a younger person has a series of dream that contain symbols of death and destruction, the symbols may indicate that the case is going in the wrong direction. The appearance of these dreams, especially if physical symptoms are not improving, may be a strong signal that a new remedy or a different type of therapy is needed On the other hand, such dreams in an older person may be indicative of a profound healing process. In the later stage of life, these symbols very well may indicate the appropriate and much needed breaking down or death of the ego, but in a younger person, they may indicate an unhealthy degenerative process.

Children's Dreams

Children often dream about their parents' problems. The more naive and innocent the children are, the more they are under the influence of the collective unconscious or may absorb the unconscious problems of their parents. Jung once analyzed a man for four weeks through his son's dreams. After the man became more conscious, the son ceased to dream of his father's problems.

Children's dreams are often a combination of simple, childlike imagery and the unconscious atmosphere of the family, along with a deep connection to the collective unconscious through archetypal symbolism. Here, archetypes from timeless ancestral energy mingle with a complicated sum of hereditary factors. These are dreams that may shape one's destiny.

Sometimes it is not only a dream, but also the inextinguishable memory of a real experience, that elicits early on, in symbolic form, certain components of the personality. From a therapeutic perspective, these memories can be used like dreams, since they remain in memory only on account of their symbolic significance. They often contain symbols that represent the template of a person's entire life. This symbolism, when taken in the context of the whole case, can give valuable clues to the recurrent pattern running through the case and may indicate the appropriate remedy. In *The Symbolic Life*, Jung writes of the importance of such dreams and events from childhood, especially when they continue to recur into adulthood:

> *Recurrent dreams, especially those that repeat from childhood into adult life, usually compensate for a defect in the conscious attitude or date from a traumatic event that has caused some particular attitude. It may also anticipate an important future issue. In any event, the recurrent dream contains important symbolism about an unresolved issue that has been following the individual for many years and will stop once that issue has been resolved.*[4]

Dreams in Provings

The question that occurs in discussing the use of dreams in homeopathic practice is, How do we use the wealth of information on dreams that is the result of remedy provings? As we have seen, the dream must be taken in the context of the individual dreamer, considering both the patient's constitution and the circumstances of his or her life. Therefore, dreams found in the repertory and materia medica must be considered in light of the whole case and are often more of a confirmation than a guiding symptom.

Let us take the following dream as an example:

> *Anxious dream, he has to go perpendicularly down into an abyss, whereupon he wakes, but retains the dangerous place so vividly in his imagination (especially when he shuts his eyes) that he remains for a long time in great fear about it and cannot calm himself.*[5]

This dream is from Hahnemann's proving of *China officinalis,* the first substance that was proved by the master of homeopathy. On a purely archetypal level, the dream seems to hint at moving down into the area of the unconscious, a feat that frightens the dreamer. What is missing, however, is certain information about the dreamer. What is left unanswered is whether or not the dream is typical of the prover before he began proving the remedy and the significance of the dream to the individual. If we had this information, we could more easily decipher the significance of the dream in the proving.

If the dream were one that the prover had dreamed many times before, it would be a symptom that belonged to the dreamer, not the remedy. Thus, in modern provings, it is important that the prover's dreams be followed for a few weeks before the proving begins and to inquire whether a dream experienced during a proving is typical of the prover or not. Only dreams that are different than the usual dreams are an effect of the remedy being proved.

If each prover is also asked to analyze the dreams using the process of association, the dreams in the provings are more likely to be meaningful in terms of understanding the themes of the remedy. Failing to do so means missing out on information that may have given us greater insight into the remedy.

Precautions

When we first begin to contact the unconscious, we are like children who see frightening ghosts in the shadows of their room at night or are afraid of what is hiding under the bed. But, just as the nighttime ghosts are created by the imagination of the child, our perception of the unconscious as being full of dark and dangerous things is created by what we put there through our conscious attitude. We must, however, respect our own resistance and any resistance that the patient has to exploring dreams. Resistance is there for a reason and, as long as we respect this response, there is little to fear from working with dreams.

The following precautions apply much more to psychoanalysis than they do to homeopathic treatment but are useful guides for homeopaths, whether or not they work with dreams. The initial interview is often an exercise in free association for patients and can lead them quite deeply into their psyche, even if they never tell dreams.

The therapist should tread more lightly with some people. These include people who have a highly charged psychic terrain as part of their spiritual structure. These people are happy to work with their dreams, but the therapist may find them to be more than he or she can handle. These people may have dreams that are "all over the place," and it is sometimes a struggle to make sense of them in a useful way. This is rarely dangerous but can be very confusing. If these people are already inundated with unconscious material, they need to focus more on the outside world rather than their dreams. In these cases, the use of dreams is counterindicated. This does not mean that a dream cannot be used to find the remedy; it simply means that the ongoing use of dream analysis should be discouraged.

Another situation that requires caution is one in which the patient is very tense because he or she is struggling to maintain sanity. These people will show themselves through extreme resistance to understanding the symbolic language of dreams. In these cases, it is especially important to respect this resistance. Resistance to moving into the realm of the psyche is often experienced as not remembering dreams. When dreams are not remembered, even after an individual has the intention of journaling his or her dreams, it is a sign of resistance, and no attempt should be made to try to alter the situation. Sometimes, however, the appropriate homeopathic remedy will stimulate healing, so that the resistance is no longer necessary and dreams will begin to be remembered.

On rare occasions, one will encounter an individual who has a great deal of negativity at the bottom of the psyche. In these cases, the deeper you go with the individual, the worse they get. This may occur in long-term chronically depressed patients or in those with very low self-esteem. The antidote is to have them focus more in the world. If this occurs during ongoing follow-up sessions, the homeopath should focus on exercise, diet, and social events. The presence of many deep and disturbing dreams after the administration of a remedy may also indicate that the remedy affected this deeply negative level of the psyche and a more superficial remedy or one that addresses the negativity must be given.

As mentioned previously, younger people need to focus more on the outside world. If you bring them into the symbolic dream world, they may stay there, languishing in the world of fantasy instead of developing relationships and a career.

The goal of working with dreams in homeopathy is to help the homeopath to gather information on which to prescribe and to follow the healing process. If people are rigidly locked into their situation in the world, working with the symbolic world of dreams and symbols will help them become more fluid and creative. People who are already inundated with material from the unconscious need more of the structure that the physical world provides. In either case, the material from dreams that is reported in the initial interview may provide a hint, not only to what remedy is needed but to what extent the homeopath should proceed in terms of dream work. In any case, the homeopath should never override a client's resistances to dream work, as these resistances are there for a reason. When a client's resistances are not honored, dream work may open up psychological material that neither the client nor the homeopath is ready to handle.

The attitude of the homeopath is another cause for concern in dream analysis. These concerns apply to the homeopathic process in general, but as we are discussing dreams, we will limit ourselves to this more specific topic. The main precaution in dream analysis is that the interpreter stays out of the picture as much as possible. This is more difficult than it seems, as it is very easy to project one's own desires and aversions onto the patient's dreams. We can also maintain a particular belief system or prejudice that will force the individual to see his or her dreams in a particular light. Even if the individual has a strong sense of self and does not comply with our belief system, our prejudice may still have a negative impact, keeping the patient from understanding the dreams in the light of his or her own unique wholeness.

In order to illustrate the impact that one person's psyche can have on another, let us turn to an encounter that Jung had when telling his dreams to Freud. Jung had had a very complicated dream of a house with many floors, each floor descending into the past as it descended below ground. As he prepared to work on the dream with Freud, he realized what Freud's view of the dream would be and what resistances the old man would have to the dream. Jung felt that a discussion about one of the rooms that contained old bones would trigger Freud's fear that Jung was anticipating and in some way wishing for his mentor's early death.

Jung thought the dream was a time line of his entire life but was afraid to tell the whole dream to Freud for fear of losing his friendship. He therefore lied to Freud about the meaning of the dream. Jung wrote:

> *Feeling quite uncertain about my own psychology, I almost auto-matically told him a lie about my "free associations" in order to escape the impossible task of enlightening him about my very personal and utterly different constitutions. I soon realized that Freud was seeking some incompatible wish of mine. And so I suggested tentatively that the skulls might refer to certain members of my family whose death, for some reason, I might desire. This proposal met with his approval, but I was not satisfied with such a "phony" solution.*[6]

If these two great minds of psychoanalysis could get into such a mess, one can imagine the possibilities for more everyday encounters. This passage also illustrates the dangers of people telling their dreams to friends and colleagues, but the main point is to show how strongly prejudices affect the telling and interpretation of dreams. It was after Jung became aware of the effect of Freud's psychic state on his whole reality that he became aware of the difficulties of dream analysis and how much depends upon the relationship and differences between the analyst and the client. As Jung defined the problem, "Dream analysis on this level is less a technique than a dialectical process between two personalities. If it is handled as a technique, the peculiarity of the subject as an individual is excluded and the therapeutic problem is reduced to the simple question: who will dominate whom?" He concluded, "For the first time it dawned on me that before we construct general theories about man and his psyche we should learn a great deal more about the real human being, rather than an abstract idea about *Homo sapiens.*"[7]

The Importance of Individualization

Dreams are a communication from the deeper unconscious level of the psyche to the more conscious aspect of the mind. They can be of help in the healing process and can assist the homeopath in finding a remedy. As we have seen, the most important and often the most difficult part of working with dreams is to avoid filtering those messages through the colors of our own perception. The dream is pointing the way toward a path that has never before been experienced by human consciousness. The path is unique, surprising, and its particular form and outcome are essentially unknown.

The challenge for those who wish to assist individuals in their healing is to know as much as possible about our healing art—and then forget it all so that we can face each situation in all its uniqueness, with a beginner's mind.

Symbolic Materia Medica

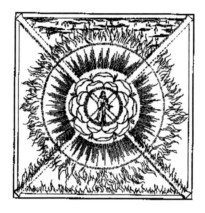

Harmonious Conception of the Light of Nature.
From which you can deduce the restoration and renovation of all things emblematic.[1]

Symbolic materia medica is an attempt to understand the relationship between substances and human consciousness. It is also meant to enrich the homeopathic materia medica with the ancient knowledge inherent within mythology and archetypal symbols. Combined with information from provings and clinical use, knowledge of the archetypal significance of the substance can help expand our understanding of the curative effect of remedies.

Hahnemann has said it is essential to perceive what needs to be healed in the individual and to match what needs to be healed to a remedy that can cure those symptoms. Finding the correct remedy according to this formula is a bit like matching shapes to a board with shapes cut out. When we work with archetypal symbolism and its relationship to human suffering, we begin to work with universal forces that are much larger than what we are able to understand. We are still, however, able to perceive the shape or symbol that is activated. Similarly, if we understand the archetypal significance in a remedy, we can match that shape to the form created by the gestalt of physical and mental symptoms within an individual.

Symbolism steers us to possibilities that are beyond what we can understand with the intellect alone. The fact that there are myths about a particular substance, a tree for instance, is interesting in itself. What is fascinating is when the same theme appears in many different cultures over thousands of years. And when these motifs appear in the provings of these substances, we are privy to a very special experience. Through these provings and our understanding of the language of symbols we learn the relationship between psyche and substance.

This symbolic materia medica is meant to enrich, not substitute for, the information in the homeopathic material contained in our traditional materia medica. Provings are the basis of understanding what a substance can cause and cure; therefore, knowledge of homeopathic remedies from provings is essential for using the following symbolic information.

The ability to take the linear information from the provings and fluidly move from the constraints of conscious logical thinking into the vastness of the symbolic realm and then return once more to logical analysis of the anamnesis, or case history, is of utmost importance in homeopathy.

Knowledge of the archetypal significance of a substance may help us in this process by opening our minds to new possibilities. It may also help us understand a significant healing potential within a remedy that has not yet been revealed because the proving was done with only a few people or at a time when people were less aware of their psychic state. Information about the symbolic use of substances may also help us to understand and organize the information that we already have. This is especially important in the case of the very well known polychrests, remedies with many uses. Finally, this knowledge helps to break the chains of culture-bound views—especially the socially oriented prejudices toward women that often appear in our materia medica—and move us to a more comprehensive understanding of the remedy.

Archetypal symbolism can also act as a guide to help us remember the remedy, because the symbol compacts information into story form, forming visual pictures that help us to remember the soul of the remedy. Given the thousands of substances used in homeopathy, this is an important factor to aid homeopaths in their practice.

I have attempted to organize this material in a way that makes it accessible and useful to the homeopath without compromising the open-ended nature of the subject. Unlike most materia medica, this one contains information on mythology and symbolism of the substance in general, as in, for instance, the general symbolism of trees, as well as in the specific remedies.

CHAPTER ELEVEN

Trees

The Archetypal Tree

The symbolic association to the tree is deeply embedded in the human psyche and is present in the religious symbolism of almost every culture, from the Amazonian rain forest to the Siberian tundra. The concept of the world tree or cosmic tree is present not only in the spiritual beliefs of societies centered around shamanism but also in Christianity, Judaism, and Buddhism as well. The grandeur and longevity of trees have inspired awe and thoughts of immortality for thousands of years.

In many indigenous societies, the tree symbolically connects the upper world, representing the heavens; the middle or the earth world; and the lower world, representing the regions below the earth realms. The cosmic tree or axis tree was revered and worshipped by the general society and used by the shaman to journey from the middle realm into the upper and lower realms. These journeys were used to gain information for the benefit of the community. Often a shaman would move through the tree to help someone who was ill or to predict where the village needed to make important changes, like planting crops or preparing for bad weather.

The cosmic tree was thought to extend from below and through the earth and up into the heavens, where it broke through the canopy of the sky at a point where the light of the gods could stream down. This symbolism persists to this day in the form of the Christmas tree, with its star shining on the very top. The lights of the Christmas tree represent the galaxies of stars as they revolve around the polestar. Little do we know as we wrap our presents and celebrate what has become a family event that we are utilizing an archetypal symbol that permeates into the depths of human consciousness.

In his yoga sutras, Patanjali tells us that meditation on the polestar will bring knowledge of the cosmos. The steadfastness of the polestar on top of the cosmic tree, with its shining lights of galaxies of stars, is considered to give the mind the stillness to comprehend the nature of the universe.

The early Celtic nature worshipers or Druids held ceremonies in sacred groves of trees. Like many other indigenous societies, they also held trees to represent the cosmic axis joining the three worlds of air, the earth, and the underworld that was the source of all water.

The tree appears in Christianity as the tree of knowledge in the garden of paradise. Adam and Eve's fall from paradise for eating the tree's fruit is similar to many earlier stories associating the world tree with separation from wholeness.

A major symbolic tree in Buddhism is the bodhi tree, a tree under which an individual reaches enlightenment. Gautama Buddha is thought to have realized his awakening under *Ficus religiosa*. All members of the Ficus family are empty inside, lacking the hard inner pith, a perfect analogy for the unencumbered state of the Buddha mind. Dr. Sarat Chandra Ghose of India did a small proving of *Ficus religiosa*. We know very little about the mental symptoms caused by this remedy; the proving contains only two. One symptom is quiet and disinclination to move, an apt symptom for a tree under which the Buddha sat in complete stillness for forty days and forty nights.

Jung spoke of the tree as a symbol of the process of growth toward the Self and the cross section of the tree as a mandala representing the Self. He associated the archetypal image of the tree with growth, nourishment, and unfolding of the individual, both physically and spiritually. In *Alchemical Studies* he writes of the tree as representing growth from below upward and from above downwards and finally being rooted to the spot in old age, personality, and finally death and rebirth.[1]

A general theme that runs through all cultures is the tree as mediator between heaven and Earth, light and dark, good and evil. With its roots buried deep within the earth and its lofty crown reaching toward heaven, the tree becomes the connection between darkness and light, integrating three different realms of life into one living plant. It symbolizes the possibility of integrating the three realms and the opposites and becoming whole. But in this world, even the lofty goal of such integration can be distorted, causing the tree of life to become the tree of death. Overzealous attempts at reaching psychic heights or delving into the depths of the underworld can leave the adventurer in a very dangerous place. Trees reach up to heaven, but they can also be struck by lightning.

In one of his stays in the asylum at Saint-Rémy, Vincent van Gogh painted *The Garden of Saint-Paul's Hospital*. It shows a tree that had been split by lightning. Van Gogh described this painting in a letter to Émile Bernard:

> *The nearest tree has an enormous trunk but has been struck by light-ning and sawn off. However, a branch still juts high up into the air and sends down a rain of dark green needles. This somber giant–with its hurt pride–contrast, if you were to lend it human characteristics, with the pale smile of a last rose on the fading bush in front of it. Under the big trees, empty stone benches, mournful little box trees, the sky is re-flected–yellow–in a puddle after the rain. A ray of sun turns the dark ochre into orange with its last reflection. Small black figures wander here and there among the tree trunks.*
>
> *Of course, you realize that the combination of red, ochre, green dark-ened with grey and the black stripes indicating the contours arouses that anguished feeling, the so-called "black-and-reds," with which some of my fellow patients are afflicted. Moreover, the motif of the great tree, struck by lightning, the wane pink-green smile of the last autumn flower, serve to reinforce this impression.*[2]

When viewing original of this painting, one is impressed with how pow-erfully van Gogh was able to portray himself and his dilemma through symbolism. He has painted the tree of death, very similar to the truncated tree emitting a ray of red light described in some early alchemical texts. Understanding this symbolism, it is no surprise that van Gogh died less than a year after finishing it.

Of all trees, the conifer is most often likened to the world tree and the *axis mundi*, or world's center. Because conifers stay green year-round, they are also associated with longevity and immortality. The Taoist Immortals were said to eat only pine kernels, needles, and resin and had no need for any other nourish-ment. This made their bodies light and able to fly. In Japanese art, conifers symbolized the life force, and in everyday life, they were an omen of good fortune. Asa Hershoff and David Warkentin, in a lecture on the conifers as homeopathic remedies, discussed the following themes related to this group of trees: feeling alone in the world, the need to be self-reliant, sensation of empti-ness inside, growing upward toward God, and a sense of duality and floating.

From the symbolism associated with trees in general, I believe that some of these themes may belong to all remedies made from trees, especially the idea of growing upward toward God. The theme of spiritual attainment appears repeatedly in mythology and symbolism associated with trees.

After researching the repertory for rubrics or symptom listings that contain many tree remedies, a few symptoms emerged. The symptoms that were most striking had to do with alcoholism. This is not surprising, since alcoholism is known to be a disease whose main cure is through spiritual attainment. It was Jung, by the way, who was instrumental in conveying this message to the person who eventually started Alcoholics Anonymous.

Dreams of trees that first appear in early childhood or that recur are a hint for the homeopath to consider a remedy that is made from a tree, especially if the individual has life issues that are connected with the general tree themes, such as an imbalanced desire for spiritual growth or integration of good and evil. A helpful exercise is to have the dreamer draw the actual tree from the dream, to further delineate what kind of tree is indicated. Even in the most rudimentary drawing, it's easy to see the difference between a palm, conifer, or deciduous tree. With this information, the homeopath can more easily explore the many homeopathic remedies made from trees to see if one of them may be the simillimum. Although we have some very well know remedies from trees, such as *Nux vomica, Ignatia, Thuja,* and *China,* most of the tree remedies are hardly proven, and many of them are underutilized.

AGATHIS AUSTRALIS
KAURI

Agathis australis, or kauri, is a giant conifer native to New Zealand. It is truly an ancestral tree, thought to have appeared on this planet over 130 million years ago. A single tree can live up to two thousand years and grow to a height of over a hundred feet. Kauri were once logged to the point where they are now endangered. Misha Norland proved this grandfather tree as a homeopathic remedy between 1993 and 1995, with twenty-eight provers.

The kauri plays an important part in the sacred creation story of the Maori, the indigenous people of New Zealand, The story points to the kauri as the world tree, standing between heaven and Earth, but in the beginning there was no separation between the two. Here is the story:

> *In the beginning there was nothingness and all was dark. The sky god joined with the earth goddess and created the land. They had many children, who were shapeless and lived in darkness because their parents were still joined together. Finally, the children tired of all this darkness and decided that something must be done about their parents, for their parents were joined together and no light could come between them.*

The fiercest of the offspring, who was also the guardian of war, wanted to kill them. However, the guardian of the forest suggested that it was better to separate them. He suggested separating the father so the sky would be far overhead, but to allow the mother to remain as close as a nursing mother.

Slowly, as slowly as the kauri tree grows, the guardian of the forest rose between the earth and the sky. He placed his shoulders against his mother, the earth, and his feet against his father, the sky, and after a long, long time the earth and the sky began to separate.

All of the children of the earth and the sky cried out, thinking that their parents were being killed, but with all of his strength, which was the strength of growth, the guardian of the forest thrust the sky upward and held him there. The guardian's body was stretched and taut as he slashed the bonds that bound his parents, and their blood spilled out upon the earth. Today this is known as kokowai, *the sacred red earth. As soon as the guardian of the forest was finished, a multitude of creatures emerged who had never known light.*

And now, the kauri stands in memory of that time, with his roots in the ground and his huge trunk reaching high up into the sky, where his branches open up into heaven.[3]

This story represents not only the creation of the world but, as with many sacred stories, it also symbolizes a phase in the individual path of development. In infancy, we are in a state of complete merging, a state of oneness with everything we experience. There is no differentiation between the self and the experience of the outside world. We must create a separation if we are to mature. The separation from this oneness is the creation of an individual sense of self, a self that we call ego. This parting from the wholeness of infancy is painful, as in the myth, and we don't want to do it. It is, however, an essential step in human development. Later, we must put the parts together and create a new type of wholeness, but the first step is the separation.

Some themes that emerged in the proving for *Kauri* directly relate to the desire to stay in this oneness. An essential theme is "longing for things lost." Most of the provers experienced a feeling of euphoria and exuberance, giggling and light floating feelings. Many of them experienced yearning for childhood and old memories. These symptoms are a sign of the longing for the oneness and the euphoric feelings that come from early connection to wholeness.

The proving also reveals many associations to water; there were dreams of water, swimming pools, lakes, waterfalls, and the sea. There were also symptoms of increased urination—some provers experiencing "everlasting pees."[4] Water itself often symbolizes the state of undifferentiated consciousness typical of pre-ego development, but these watery symptoms also allude to another aspect of mythology surrounding the kauri. An ancient Maori myth tells of the association of the kauri and the whale. As the story goes, the whale and the kauri, each being giants of their own realm, admired one another and became friends. But the whale could not leave his watery realm to join the kauri, and the kauri could not leave the land. As a way of expressing their friendship, they exchanged skins. The whale took off its gray skin and gave it to the kauri, and the kauri took off its skin and gave it to the whale.

The whale is mentioned in many creation myths as both the upholder of the cosmos and the container of the multitude of opposites, similar to the alchemists' representation of undifferentiated wholeness, the Mercurial fountain. As in the story of Jonah and the whale, and many other initiatory myths, the whale also represents both the vehicle for the hero's journey and the trials and tribulations the hero must endure in order to complete the journey.

The sacred story and proving of *Kauri* show us the connection between this ancient world tree and the process of growth from undifferentiated wholeness into individuation. Given these indications, this ancient tree remedy is likely to help those who are looking backward to have the courage to separate from an earlier stage of development and to move forward into maturity.

Brosimum Utile
COW TREE

Known as the cow tree, *Brosimum utile* grows in the rain forest on the Atlantic coast of Costa Rica and southward into Columbia and Ecuador. Attaining a height of up to a hundred feet and living more than two hundred years, this tree exudes a milklike sap that is used by the local herbalists to treat indigestion and stomach ulcers. The sap is also said to taste like cream when fresh and is sometimes used to lighten coffee.

I gathered a specimen on a trip to Costa Rica in 1998, and Michael Quinn, of Hahnemann Pharmacy in California, prepared a remedy. A proving was done, double-blind, with eight provers and eight supervisors from the Five Elements School of Classical Homeopathy from 1998 to 1999 and was supervised by my associate, Deborah Ford, who was not told what substance we were proving. The supervisors recorded symptoms and dreams of the provers for two weeks before the proving and proceeded according to standardized guidelines, as developed by Jeremy Sherr.

I was interested in this tree because of the milklike sap and because, after spending a month in the rain forest, I became intimately aware of the interdependence of all of the plants and animals. If one large tree is cut down, many other species die because of the disturbance of the ecosystem. I hoped that the proving would bring some insight into the relationship of all beings, not only within the rain forest but the within the entire planet. As the rain forest is a net of interdependent species, so is this planet dependent upon the rain forest for maintaining the integrity of its many ecosystems.

The milklike sap is a direct connection to the mythological tie between trees and the mother goddess. The Yakuts of northern Siberia believe that there is, at the "golden navel of the Earth," a tree with eight branches; and, there, the first man was born. He feeds on the milk of a woman who half emerges from the trunk of the tree.[5]

As soon as the proving began, there were a lot of problems. Most of the provers did not want to communicate with their supervisors. There was a lot of secrecy and isolation. One prover locked herself in the bathroom when her husband came home from work. The most pervasive symptom was apathy. Unfortunately, the proving extended over Christmas and spoiled that holiday for a lot of families. One usually very responsible prover didn't put up her tree until the day after Christmas.

Although not officially a proving symptom, it was noted that many of the supervisors had symptoms of procrastination, and one student found it so unpleasant to be around the remedy because of the isolation, depression, and procrastination that she buried the remedy in her back yard. Everyone hated how he or she felt on the remedy and seemed to be affected by just being around it. The remedy didn't seem to remain in its bottle but had a very heavy, permeating energy that was impossible to contain. I can understand why one person felt they had to bury it.

Here are some of the main proving symptoms:

MIND: Wanting to escape or retreat, not wanting be bothered with anything. Apathy.
Separation, isolation, hating being married. Desire to be left alone.

Dealing with the world as a front, but I don't care most of the time.

Refuses to speak (answer). Desire to hide from people. Secretive. Weeping.

DREAMS: Sex, he is superhuman, dancing, breasts, animals (deer), flying an airplane, trees.

HEAD: Headache.

FACE: Eruptions, pimples.

BACK: Stiffness in neck.

STOMACH: Pains, burning, sick feeling.

ABDOMEN: Gurgling intestines, cramping pain.

SEX: Desire increased.

RECTUM: Constant urging for stool, frequent stool, flatulence.

The proving of the tree shows the pattern of isolation and indifference that keeps us from experiencing a deep connection with one another. The dreams reveal the other side of the story; they show the connection, the dancing, sexuality and breasts. Many provers and supervisors had dreams of animals and trees.

CINNAMONUM CAMPHORA
CAMPHORA

Cinnamonum camphora is a tree that grows up to 150 feet tall in the forests of Indochina and Japan. The remedy *Camphora,* commonly called camphor, is made from the oil of the camphor tree, which crystallizes within the wood. This white crystalline substance is burned in many Hindu ceremonies in order to purify the air. It symbolizes purity and is associated with the color white. Camphor is said to have the power of sublimation, which is the channeling of lower impulses and energies into higher, more spiritual, and creative energies and activities. The alchemists used camphor in many of their distillation processes, and oil of camphor was used against putrefaction, "fits of the mother," and "passions of the heart."

Camphor was also used in sepulchral lamps to relieve the gloom hanging over the grave, to relieve the darkness of death and the darkness of the tomb. Burning camphor was set in water, where it would continue to burn, even underwater. It is also burned as incense.

Camphor has been used as a purifying substance, most often by burning or lighting it, to assuage the forces of evil, darkness, and death and to bring in higher spiritual energies and light.

As a homeopathic remedy, the coldness, collapse, and cramping caused by *Camphora* are well known. The mental state *Camphora* creates is less understood. It is not unlike the states that the burning of camphor has been thought to assuage. Here are some excepts from the text under the heading *"Camphora"* in Allen's *Encyclopedia of Pure Materia Medica:*

> *I could not lie; the thought continually occurred, as in delirium, "I am dead! No, I am not dead! But indeed I must be dead!" and thus I flew round about myself like a top, with no other feeling than for the strong smell of the Camphor.*
>
> *What soul could paint to itself my everlasting dwelling as the Evil One, alone in a vast universe, without faith or hope, and my heart forever broken by unimaginable tortures?*
>
> *The external world existed for me no longer.... I was alone in the great universe, the last of all things. I was the final and solitary fragment of the whole creation. There was no other feeling in my soul than that of my hopeless, endless damnation.*[6]

The fears brought up in the proving of *Camphora* are deep existential fears of death, darkness, and evil—the same fears camphor has been burned to dispel for eons. The provers experienced the horror of being dead while still alive. They felt the darkness and loneliness of death and the chilling fear of evil. What *Camphora* brought out in them was what lies at the very bottom of the human mind—the thoughts that we avoid, that we deny and fear. That some day we will die and that darkness and inescapable evil exist in the world are thoughts most of us would prefer not to entertain.

Denial of the inevitability of death is so strong that, even in very old age, some cannot accept it. Jack Kornfield, who is a wonderful storyteller and vipassana teacher, tells a story of his visit to a ninety-five-year-old woman who was dying. Clinging to him, afraid of death, she exclaimed, "Why me, God?!" It takes a very strong and well-trained mind to accept the fact that death is always with us. When one can integrate the awareness that death is always just around the corner, one gains a powerful presence and ability to be in the moment. Thus the famous Sioux battle cry, "Today is a good day to die." But when the awareness of death is present at every moment and the mind is not strong enough to hold this awareness gracefully like a samurai, *Camphora* may be needed to remedy the horror of this reality.

Hahnemann wrote that in gross amounts (as opposed to the potentized remedy), camphor was an antidote for the overly strong effects of many remedies and then added an interesting warning:

> *. . . hence it must have a sort of general pathological action, which,*
> *however, we are unable to indicate by any general expression; nor can we*
> *even attempt to do so for fear of straying into the domain of shadows,*
> *where knowledge and observation cease, while imagination deceives us*
> *into accepting dreams as truth; where we, in short, abandoned by the*
> *guiding of plain experience, grope about in the dark, and with every*
> *desire to penetrate into the inner essence of things, about which little*
> *minds so presumptuously dogmatize, we gain nothing by such hyper-*
> *physical speculations but noxious error and self deception.*[7]

This leads one to wonder if Hahnemann is warning about looking into the deeper meaning of camphor because he truly believed that such explorations were of no use, or if he was, at that moment, proving the substance. His statement, although typical of Hahnemann, is strongly tinged with the fear of darkness and unknown that is voiced by the provers of this remedy.

After writing this section, I was surprised to find that *Camphora* had also affected me. I had been writing until late in the evening, and on going to sleep, I had a dream about death that was so violent and frightening it woke me up. Uncharacteristically, I stayed awake for many hours feeling a sense of fear and apprehension, listening to things that go "bump in the night."

My dream had within it images and situations that were characteristic of my individual complexes, but it was also, like Hahnemann's words above, tinged with the qualities of evil and death brought out by *Camphora*. In every proving, there is this combination of that which belongs to the individual and that which belongs to the substance. This is also true in understanding the archetypal significance of a substance. There is the essence of the archetype and the meaning that it has for the individual person. The art of homeopathy requires that the homeopath is able to match what the remedy can cure to what needs to be healed in the individual.

THEOBROMA CACAO
CHOCOLATE

Ah, chocolate, food of the gods, the sacred drink of the Aztecs. No one needs to tell us why it was named the food of the gods, when we allow this delight to sweetly melt in our mouths. The Aztec nobility drank chocolate as a thick beverage and treasured it as an aphrodisiac. Casanova was said to drink chocolate before his adventures, and the use of chocolate as a love offering is well known. However, as we shall see, the essence of chocolate as a remedy goes beyond sexual and romantic love.

The cacao tree, *Theobroma cacao*, which grows to a height of twenty to thirty-five feet, is usually planted in hot, humid areas with heavy rainfall. The tree is very delicate when it is young and must be shaded from the hot sun. For this reason, the seedlings are planted beneath large shade trees of different species (often in the Leguminosae family) known as *"Madre de cacao."*

There are two provings of chocolate in our materia medica. One is of *Cocoa*, the powdered cocoa bean, and is mentioned in Allen's *Encyclopedia of Pure Materia Medica*. *Cocoa* was not proved in potency, but by drinking the actual cocoa in hot water. The more recent and thorough proving was done by Jeremy Sherr and the Dynamis School with the "best quality Belgium dark chocolate" potentized into a homeopathic remedy.

The following is an Andean myth about cocoa that may give us further insight into the essence of chocolate as a healing substance.

> *A long time ago there was an omnipotent deity named Sibu who could grow animals and humans from seeds. One day, Sibu gave all of his precious seeds to another deity, Sura, with instructions on how to use them for the benefit of all. Sura, having something else to do, buried the seeds in the ground and left. While he was away, a trickster deity named Jabaru dug up all the seeds and ate them, leaving nothing for the creation-work of Sibu and Sura. When Sura returned, the trickster Jabaru slit Sura's throat and buried him where the seeds had been. Very pleased with himself, Jabaru left the scene and went home to his wives.*
>
> *Many moons later, the trickster Jabaru passed by where Sura was buried and saw that two strange trees had sprung up from his grave: a cacao tree and a calabash. The omnipotent deity Sibu stood quietly beside the trees. Sibu asked the trickster to brew him a cup of cocoa from the tree. Jabaru agreed and picked a bean-filled pod and a calabash fruit and took them to his wives, who brewed the cocoa and filled the hollowed out calabash shell with the rich drink. When the trickster Jabaru returned with the cocoa, Sibu politely insisted, "No, you drink first." Jabaru complied eagerly, gulping down the delicious drink as fast as he could. However, his delight soon changed to agony as the cocoa caused his belly to swell and swell until it burst wide open, spilling the stolen seeds all over the ground. Sibu then restored his friend Sura to life and returned the seeds to him so that all humans and animals might one day grow from those precious seeds and enjoy Earth's bounty.*[8]

In his proving of chocolate, Jeremy Sherr mentions a Mexican legend of Quetzalcoatl, the Toltec and Aztec god of the wind and air, who journeyed into the land of the lost paradise of the sun god and brought back the cacao seeds. He planted the seeds in his garden and, inebriated with the cocoa liquor, inspired disciples and taught them the arts of agriculture, astronomy, and medicine. Quetzalcoatl later became the ruler of Mexico.

These two myths of cacao show how the drinking of cocoa is associated with the development of civilization. In the Andean myth, cocoa overcomes greed by breaking open the belly of the trickster who had eaten all of the seeds. In the Mexican legend, inebriation by cocoa inspires Quetzalcoatl to teach the arts of civilization to the Mexican people.

During the Dynamis School proving, one prover experienced many feelings and delusions about being a hedgehog, a symptom that was thought to relate to irritability that was seen throughout the proving. In East Africa, the hedgehog was credited with the invention of agriculture and fire. Medieval paintings portrayed the hedgehog as a symbol of greed and gluttony, based on the belief that the hedgehog rolled over fallen fruit, impaling the fruit on its spines and returning back to its home laden with fruits with which it would feed to its young. The symbol of the hedgehog leads us again to the theme of the development of civilization (here agriculture and fire) and of greed and gluttony.

Here are the words of one of the provers who had a direct experience of the theme that unfolds in the myths:

> *Thoughts about the "veneer of civilization" that inhibits how we really feel and keeps us from displaying what we're like beneath the surface. It seems a legitimate layer, but so is the layer beneath it, and I feel amused and happy to meet it. This feeling continued for a few days, a very graphic picture of a veneer—a layer of learned social behavior lifting and detaching from a basis that is thick, dark, solid, instinctual animal.*⁹

Many of the symptoms from the proving of chocolate relate to the inability to love, connect with, and nurture others. The provers felt isolated and estranged from others, wanting to be alone. The theme of not wanting to nurture children also appeared. There were delusions of being alone in the world and separated from the world. As we look at all of these symptoms in the light of the mythological motif, we begin to see a theme emerge concerning the challenge of living in a society that inhibits our deeper animal instincts in order for humankind to exist together. The thread of greed that appears in the myths and in the hoarding of chocolate and the overwhelming cravings many people have for it points toward the negative aspect of the instinctual level. The question that chocolate poses to us is, How do we live together in a civilized manner without suppressing our instinctual selves? Moreover, how do we honor our instinctual selves without succumbing to overwhelming greed?

GINKGO BILOBA
GINKGO

The ginkgo tree grows from eighty to a hundred feet tall and can live more than five hundred years (some say two thousand years). Although similar to the conifers, the ginkgo has its own botanical category. It is the sole living link between the lower and higher plants, between ferns and conifers. It is considered a "living fossil," as it is the only living survivor of the Ginkgocaceae family. One ginkgo survived the bombing of Hiroshima and still stands in Japan, just one kilometer away from the blast center of the atomic bomb explosion.

The earliest mention of *Ginkgo biloba*'s use in medicine is from around 2800 B.C., which relates a story of *Ginkgo biloba*'s discovery as a medicine. Shen Nung, a legendary emperor and sage, noticed that some members of his court were becoming quite senile in their older years. One day while the emperor was gazing at a beautiful ginkgo tree in his garden, he heard a voice whispering in his ear, saying, "The tree you are looking at will restore the minds of your friends and relatives." Knowing to trust this voice, Shen Nung instructed his head herbalist to pick some leaves from the tree and create a brew out of them. The emperor served this tea to the senile court elders, and within weeks every one of them had regained much of their lost memories.

Ginkgo has been used in Western medicine since the 1950s for weakness of memory and early symptoms of Alzheimer's disease. Ginkgo is a "vasoactivator" that improves the circulation of the blood to the brain and the body's periphery. Reportedly, ginkgo helps improve memory and alleviates vertigo and tinnitus, and extracts of ginkgo can also aid in depression and anxiety.

Ginkgo was proved in 1933 by E. A. Maury, from 1987 to 1990 by Franz Swoboda and Peter Konig, and more recently by Anne Shadde of Germany. Many symptoms associated with the remedy are consistent with the use of the herbal preparation. Provers experienced poor concentration, loss of memory, absentmindedness, and forgetfulness. They also felt everything was "too much for them" and were totally exhausted. They felt emotionally numb and apathetic, postponing everything, not even bothering to cook or eat. Finally, the provers felt very old. In other words, they felt like old, forgetful people who were becoming senile, not unlike the elderly nobles of Shen Nung's court and many contemporary senior citizens suffering from memory loss and depression.

The provers remembered their dreams clearly and, in light of the ginkgo having survived the Hiroshima bombing, it is interesting to note the theme of war and bombing found among the dreams. Provers had dreams of bomb explosions, corpses, battles, and war, of escaping, and death in the family.

Another unique quality of the ginkgo is that the tree is dioecious, meaning that there are male trees and female trees. Anne Shadde, a German homeopath who also proved the remedy *Ginkgo,* found that there was a theme of male/female, anima/animus, the searching for a soul mate, and a strong sense of the two in one in the proving. In a seminar she gave in Florida in 1998, Anne told the following legend, which may have been inspired by the ginkgo's beautiful two-lobed leaf:

> *Ginkgo was the first tree on Earth and around this tree there were just couples, men and women living in freedom and peace. Whenever they left the tree they would be cut apart. One day a big storm blew away all the couples and broke them apart. Since this time they have to search for each other. God said to the ginkgo tree, "I will give you leaves as the couples were before."*

The theme of two in one is also seen in Goethe's poem inspired by a ginkgo tree growing in his garden and dedicated to his former lover, Marianne von Willemer. In the poem, Goethe asks the question "Does it represent one living creature which has divided itself? Or are these two, which have decided that they should be as one?" Then he answers his own question saying, "That I am one and two."

Goethe understood the theme of the union of opposites seen in *Ginkgo biloba.* This theme is frequently mentioned by the alchemists and is the subject of many of Jung's writings. Jung's *Mysterium Coniunctionis,* thought to be one of his most difficult works, is about the union of opposites, as it appears both internally, in the individuation process, and in the writings of the alchemists. The alchemists expressed the union in many ways, frequently using the symbols of the unity of the sun and the moon, Sol and Luna, which in turn creates the *lapis philosophorum,* the goal of the alchemist's work.

From a psychological point of view, the union of opposites stands for the integration of the diverse aspects within an individual. One of the most important of these is the integration of the animus in a woman and the anima in the man. This results in a balance between male and female energies in one individual, an important aspect of personal growth and individuation. The individual who may possibly benefit from *Ginkgo biloba* has an overwhelming need to find a soul mate. These people have the romantic notion that all will be satisfied by finding the lost parts of oneself in another. In actuality, what is being projected out onto the world is the intense need for personal integration, the union of opposites within.

The symptoms associated with old age and memory loss are, at least partly, connected with the theme of the union of opposites. In the early part of life, the need for this type of unity on the part of the psyche is not so pressing. Other challenges, such as the development of the ego and finding one's life work is more appropriate to this time of life. However, after midlife, one has a greater need to integrate the parts of one's life that have not developed. Nature then seems to press us to delve into that which we have not explored in order to enrich ourselves with a rebirth in the second half of life. If we do not respond to this urging, what often happens is fossilization, a moving into premature senility and a decline. We see too many of our elders in this situation. Is it that they have not heeded the call toward the union of opposites? Perhaps for some of them it is not too late and they can benefit from this ancient and wise tree made into a homeopathic remedy.

TILIA EUROPAEA
LINDEN TREE

The linden tree, *Tilia europaea*, grows throughout Europe and is frequently planted in the central area of a town or settlement. Thus, this tree, which can grow to a height of up to 130 feet, has borne witness to many aspects of community life, from romantic meetings to harsh trials by town fathers. However, whether the activities of the inhabitants of its community are benign or harsh, the linden tree, or lime tree as it is often called, emits a sweet fragrance from its honey-scented blossoms.

According to Jung, the well known "village linden-tree" is clearly characterized as a mother symbol.[10] It has been associated with Freya, the most motherly of the Germanic goddesses and staunch defender of the natural realm. The myths of Freya abound with themes of caring and protecting her children and keeping the bonds of society strong.

A full report of the earliest proving of *T. europaea* is found in Allen's *Encyclopedia of Pure Materia Medica*. *T. europaea* is considered to be a hybrid of *T. platyphyllos* (large-leaved lime) and *T. cordata* (small-leaved lime). *Tilia cordata*, which is the national tree of the Czech Republic, was proved in 1996 by Robert Bannon, using a remedy prepared from the root, bark, leaf, buds, and flowers of the tree. In the Czech Republic, *Tilia cordata* is planted in front of homes, where it is thought to provide protection for the house and its inhabitants.

The linden tree is associated with many myths and legends, but an earlier legend, set in ancient Anatolia, what is now Turkey, is the story of Baucis and Philemon.

> *Once upon a time, a long time ago, Jupiter and his son Mercury came down to Earth disguised as weary travelers. They went from house to house in a particular countryside to find lodging for the night but none of the country people would open their homes to them. Finally, they came upon a humble thatched cottage, the abode of Baucis and her husband Philemon. Now Baucis and Philemon were an elderly married couple who had lived together since they were very young. Although they were very poor, they made up for their poverty with their love and kindness.*
>
> *When the strangers came to their door, Baucis and Philomen invited the strangers in and prepared a humble but delicious dinner for them. The old couple served hot stew and simple wine. For dessert there were fruits and wild honey. But most important was their friendly faces and hearty welcome.*
>
> *As they dined together, the old couple was astonished to see that the wine began to replenish itself as soon as it was poured out of the pitcher. They realized that their guests were not ordinary mortals but gods. They fell to their knees and implored the gods to forgive them the meager entertainment.*
>
> *Their heavenly guests then replied, " We are gods and this village was not kind to us. You alone will be saved from our punishment. Leave this house quickly and go to the top of the hill. Baucis and Philemon quickly*

obeyed, climbing the steep slope of the hill. When they were almost to the top they turned around and saw the entire countryside covered by a huge lake. Their home was the only one left standing. As they watched and lamented for their neighbors, their cottage turned into a temple.

Then Jupiter spoke. "Tell me what favor I can grant you for your kindness." The old couple thought and then together asked that, when it came time for them to die, that they could die together at the same hour. They had been together for so long that neither could bear to leave the other. Their wish was granted. They became the guardians of the temple, and one day when they were both very old, Baucis saw Philemon begin to grow leaves and Philemon saw Baucis begin to do the same. Then a leafy crown grew over their old heads. They barely had time to exchange their parting words. "Farewell, dear spouse," they said together, as the bark closed over their mouths.

The local shepherd still shows the two trees, a linden tree and an oak, standing side by side, made out of the two good old people.[11]

In the original proving of *Tilia europaea* recorded in Allen's *Encyclopedia of Pure Materia Medica,* we see a longing for this ideal relationship:

Lovesick; all his thoughts centered upon an ideal woman; in this reverie he was possessed by a sweet melancholy, which it was impossible to describe; every earthly sense seemed far away.

The opposite symptoms of quarrelsomeness and irritable moods are also indicated:

Irritable, critical mood, inclined to quarrel and get angry, even from the slightest difference of opinion.

The symptoms show a longing for deep relationship and yet irritability and anger, the inability to withstand any difference of opinion. The tree, with its sweet fragrance, and the story seem to be telling us of the possibility of enduring love and kindness in relationship with others; the proving gave the symptoms that need to be cured to find that love and kindness within ourselves. Let's now look at the more recent proving of *Tilia cordata.* Robert Bannan's analysis of his proving is as follows:

My analysis of the proving is that the most important feeling of the remedy is that of hopelessness, helplessness and resignation. They feel they are in a situation that is dangerous and threatening, that they have no

power and influence over the situation and are at a loss what to do.
What happens as a result of this is that they go into a non-reactive mode.
They stop feeling danger, they dissociate from the situation and from
feeling in general. This leads to feelings of being separated, cut off, of
there being a barrier between themselves and others. They feel forsaken
and isolated in a sort of dead world.[12]

The feeling of being in a dangerous and threatening situation is interest-ing in light of the connection with Freya as the mother/protector. Without this early protection, people often feel that the world is a very dangerous and threatening place and feel separate and isolated. In this state, a person is unable to live the love and kindness experienced by Baucis and Philemon. Fortunately, we are working with the law of similars, and what can cause a problem is capable of curing it.

Here we begin to see what all the myths of the linden tree are telling us. Through the collective experience of humankind with this tree, the healing properties of the tree are revealed. However, only after the proving can we more deeply understand the linden's use.

Some physical symptoms associated with this remedy are:

Profuse sweat; without relief. The more he sweats the greater the pain.
Particularly suitable for women after parturition, and for children dur-ing dentition. Heavy dragging sensation in urethra, uterus and rectum.
As if everything would fall out of pelvis."

The physical symptoms are similar to those of *Sepia,* but the feeling of the remedy is very different. The essence of *Tilia* is the longing for a deep loving relationship, while with *Sepia* there is a desire for independence.

CHAPTER TWELVE

Vines

Healing Entanglements

Like most symbols, the vine represents two opposing aspects of reality. The vine's need for support and clinging symbolize the attitudes and concepts that tie us to material life—the need to keep things unchanging in a world of constant change. On the other hand, the climbing nature of the vine, reaching up from the darkness of the forest floor into the sunlight, also symbolizes the vehicle through which humankind can reach into the abodes of the gods. Here the vine becomes the ladder upon which those seeking spiritual knowledge can ascend.

One of the few traditions in which the symbolism of the vine is represented in its dual and paradoxical nature is in Zen Buddhism. The thirteenth-century Zen master Eihei Dogen uses the imagery of twining vines to represent both blocks to understanding and the vehicle by which one can become aware of one's Buddha nature.[1]

In the former meaning, the twining vine represents words and concepts that obstruct the mind and become a hindrance to understanding the true nature of things. In the latter, the twining vine represents a path to freedom through oneness of teacher and disciple. The intertwining of the consciousness of the teacher and disciple allows for the direct transmission of knowledge. Known in Zen tradition as face-to-face transmission, this intertwining is a means by which knowledge has been passed down from master to disciple in an unbroken lineage since the time of the Buddha.

More frequently, the vine is seen as a symbol for ascension and the communication between heaven and Earth. The vine, and more particularly, the grape vine and its wine, is an important symbol in the Mandaean culture. The Mandaeans, Middle Eastern followers of Saint John the Baptist, believe that wine is the physical form of light, wisdom, and purity. The archetype of wine resided in the heavenly kingdom. Internally, the archetypal vine consisted of water; its leaves were fashioned from the spirits of light, and its nodes were seeds of light. The vine was regarded as a cosmic tree, since its branches enfolded the heavens and its clusters of grapes were the stars.

The symbolism of the vine appears in the shamanistic rites of many cultures all over the world, including the Australian, Amazonian, and Melanesian. The vine is often thought to be a means by which the shaman moves from Earth to heaven and back again.

A vine found in the Amazonian rain forest, *Banisteriopsis caapi*, is a most sacred plant for the Shipibo-Conibo people of Peru. This vine represents the center of their knowledge and influences their health and their art. They refer to it as the ladder to the Milky Way, or spirit vine. A major ingredient in the vision-producing formula ayahuasca, the plant itself is also known as ayahuasca, or "vine of the soul." The vine is considered to be the sacred mother plant that contains all the information about the medicinal and practical uses of all of the plants in the rain forest. Shamans who specialize in the use of ayahuasca ingest the formula and, through their visions, transmit the messages from the sacred plant to the people. Many of these visions are in the form of patterns that represent health, beauty, and orderliness and can be found on much of their artwork. When a member of this community is unable to see these patterns or transform them into artwork, it is considered unhealthy and is treated by the shaman.

Presently three provings of *Ayahuasca* exist, one by Nancy Herrick, another by the Irish homeopath Declan Hammond, and a meditation proving by the Prometheus Group in England.

Common symptoms of those ingesting the substance are visions, especially visions of snakes and of panthers. According to Declan Hammond, *Ayahuasca* is useful for overcoming addictions and is indicated by a feeling of being trapped in a place of terror, feeling out of the body, and lost in the universe.

In modern Western society, vines are known more as a symbol of weakness than of spiritual ascension. The clinging nature of the vine is symbolized in the contemporary expression "clinging vine," meaning an overly dependent person. Critical of dependency, this metaphor for a climbing vine no longer indicates the warm cozy feeling in the old refrain: "Cuddle up and be my little clinging vine."

Whether clinging vine or ladder to heaven, a synopsis of the symbolic meaning of the vine throughout time and in various cultures shows the paradoxical themes of desire for spiritual attainment and addiction to the material world. That the addiction is to people, love, money, or substance makes little difference; the individual remains entwined with the object of his or her addiction.

The provings and clinical information on homeopathic remedies made from vines indicate that there is a similarity between the archetypal symbolism of the vine and what the remedies can cure. Some remedies, however, lean more toward substance addiction, such as *Alcoholus* and *Ayahuasca,* and others such as *Bryonia* and *Rhus toxicodendron* are for obsession with family and material success. Concern for family and one's financial welfare are healthy concerns, when in balance, but homeopathic remedies are needed in those cases when the concern becomes obsession and affects the body as well as the mind.

Conversely, substance addiction is almost always seen as a negative; however, behind this addiction lies a need as important as financial and family relationship, that of spiritual health. The homeopathic solution lies in moving toward rather than away from what entangles us allowing that which entangles to create freedom. This is the law of similars. As Zen master Dogen writes; "Gourd vines entangle with gourd vines."[2]

ALCOHOLUS
SPIRITS OF WINE, ETHYL ALCOHOL

The remedy *Alcoholus* is made from ethyl alcohol (CH_3CH_2OH) and was proved in the physical substance by Timothy F. Allen, who consumed one and a half ounces of pure spirits of wine every day for five days. His *Encyclopedia of Pure Materia Medica* has the most extensive material on this remedy; gathered from various sources. Many of the symptoms are from observation of persons intoxicated by alcohol.

Physical and general symptoms include chronic inflammation of the eyes, acne rosacea, numbness, shocks and restlessness of the limbs, and a feeling of something lodged in the esophagus. Other symptoms include overpowering sleepiness, excessive thirst or no thirst, and aversion to or desire for alcohol.

One modern proving was done in Holland. This proving showed secret drinking and the shame that is also noted in Allen's materia medica.

The mental symptoms caused by alcohol show an extremely labile state of mind. One moment there are sweet outpourings of friendship, the next the drinker is abusive and cursing, mocking his or her friends. The drinker can feel transported into a garden of pleasure, seeing only cheerful and agreeable objects, but the predominating feeling is love and desire. However, fear of misfortune; unaccountable, vague fear, and melancholy with inclination to commit suicide are also experienced. The drinker might feel courageous or fearful, with fear becoming an abyss. Or the drinker may feel insulted or pursued by murderers robbers, or the police.

Alcohol may cause overpowering sleepiness, but solitude and repose in bed may increase the drinker's anxiety. Due to this anxiety, the person refuses to remain in bed and must leave the house. He or she divulges all secrets and exposes all of his or her weaknesses. The drinker is boisterous, talkative. He or she craves attention and laughs too much, and can be very cruel and unmanageable. The drinker may destroy things.

This is the chaotic life of the alcoholic and, to some degree, those who are touched by alcohol through their heredity. This state of changeableness, the dichotomy between love and hate and lack of control can be even more devastating for those who are in its grips without imbibing.

Children of alcoholics or those with a history of alcoholism in the family are many times restless, overactive, and tend to lie. The French homeopath and pediatrician Didier Grandgeorge recommends *Alcoholus* for such children. These children may crave attention and go to great lengths to receive it. They can be little performers, laughing, dancing, and telling great stories in order to be center stage. But this can all shift, and they can become unmanageable, having temper tantrums or becoming destructive. Because of the overwhelming desire for attention, along with the sudden destructive acts, the homeopath could easily confuse this state with the state indicating the need for *Tarentula Hispanica* and a careful differential must be made. When *Tarentula* gives good results but stops working in these cases, *Alcoholus* should be considered.

Alcoholus should also be considered in children or adults who were born to an alcoholic mother. Heavy drinking of alcohol or drinking at all at critical points during pregnancy can lead to fetal alcohol syndrome, a problem that affects 1 in every 750 babies in the United States. Even babies without a full diagnosis of this syndrome, which includes mental retardation and central nervous system impairment, may still have the syndrome. Even babies with normal intellectual abilities may exhibit impulsivity, hyperactivity, learning and attention difficulties, developmental delays, and motor problems because of exposure to alcohol in the womb. An individual may exhibit one, many, or all of these symptoms.

Given the health problems connected with the imbibing of the "fruit of the vine" and the difficulty of giving up the habit for those who are addicted to it, there must be a powerful psychological reason why the drinking and abuse of alcohol persists all over the world.

Alcoholics Anonymous has been one of the most successful programs to help alcoholics deal with their problem. The basic tenant of AA, that alcoholism is a spiritual disease, is an idea that was inspired by Carl Jung. Bill W., cofounder of Alcoholics Anonymous, was with Jung when he commented that the situation of a particular alcoholic, Rowland H., was hopeless unless he could have a true spiritual or religious awakening. These remarks subsequently led to Bill W.'s spiritual awakening and cure. This in turn resulted in his founding of Alcoholics Anonymous in 1934.

In 1961, Bill W. wrote Jung a letter acknowledging Jung's deep perception of the plight of the alcoholic. Jung's reply not only shows his belief in the connection between alcoholism and the need for a spiritual experience but also, astonishingly, describes the cure as a simillimum:

> *His [Rowland H.] craving for alcohol was the equivalent, on a low level, of the spiritual thirst of our being for wholeness, expressed in medieval language: the union with God.*
>
> *How could one formulate such an insight in a language that is not misunderstood in our days?*
>
> *The only right and legitimate way to such an experience is that it happens to you in reality, and it can only happen to you when you walk on a path which leads you to a higher understanding. . . .*
>
> *You see, "alcohol" in Latin is spiritus, and you use the same world for the highest religious experience as well as for the most depraving poison. The helpful formula therefore is: spiritus contra spiritum.*[3]

The symbolism of alcohol, and particularly wine, shows both the dichotomy of the symptoms found in the materia medica of *Alcoholus* and the quest for spiritual union described by Jung. Dionysus, the god of wine, is perhaps the most well known of these symbols. Also known as Bacchus, he is associated with a drunken and orgiastic nature religion and was the only Olympian god born of a mortal mother. He contains within himself the paradox of being both human and divine and spans the realms of blissful ecstasy and wild and bloody savagery. He is shown as a beautiful young man crowned with ivy and grape leaves and dressed only in a leopard skin, carrying a wine cup.

Dionysian orgies were filled with drinking and dancing and inspired the participants into ecstatic states and experiences of transformation. These orgies could also be violent and terrifying, with the sacrifice of animals and eating of raw flesh and drinking of blood. The eating of raw animals has been described as a kind of communion in which Dionysus's worshippers feast on the god. Later, this was changed to the drinking of wine, which was seen as the blood of Dionysus.

In spite of their violent side, the ultimate purpose of these rituals was to destroy inhibitions and give expression to that which the soul needed to be liberated. The cult of Dionysus demonstrates the effort that is needed and the lengths to which human beings will go to break through barriers separating them from the divine.

As the god of wine, intoxication, and creative ecstasy, Dionysus symbolizes the attempt to achieve spiritual ecstasy and divine inspiration from plant life, just as imbibers of wine attempt to attain spiritual ecstasy in their cups. The dichotomy between this need and the violence wrought by alcohol is mirrored in the remedy *Alcoholus*, with its visions of peace and feelings of love contrasted sharply with violence and abusive and destructive behavior. *Alcoholus* is a remedy that deserves more study, and it should be added to the list of remedies that may be helpful for those with the disease or with a family history of alcoholism.

BRYONIA ALBA
WILD HOPS

Bryonia is one of our early homeopathic remedies, having been proved by Hahnemann and used since his time for many acute diseases. It is most frequently used for treatment of colds, flu, and injuries, where there is irritability, a desire to remain motionless, and great dryness and thirst. *Bryonia* is also an important remedy for bronchitis and pneumonia.

Along with its usefulness in acute diseases, *Bryonia* is also a remedy for more chronic problems, when the indicated for the whole person. The *Bryonia* personality is focused on the material plane, extremely concerned and even anxious over business matters. He or she is very down to earth, not interested in creativity or in spiritual pursuits. With little imagination, reliable and methodical, these people even dream of business and may spend a great deal of time in the homeopathic interview speaking of finances and business. They have a great deal of anxiety and fear about financial security. Of the twenty remedies listed under fear of poverty in the *Complete Repertory*, *Bryonia* is the only one in bold type, indicating this symptom to the highest degree.

In other words, the world of people needing *Bryonia* revolves around money and material matters to which they cling tightly for support and security. They may also cling tightly to their homes and are often hesitant to travel any distance. When these people are away, they have a desire to return home.

This behavior is very similar to the plant white bryony, or wild hops, from which the remedy is made. White bryony is a climbing vine that has long tendrils that extend from the stem in search of some support. On finding a support, the tendril curls around it first in a clockwise direction and then in the counterclockwise direction, providing an extremely stable support for the plant.

If we look more deeply into this matter, we will see that this theme of clinging to the outer, material world is expanded in the historical use of the root of the plant. The remedy is made from the plant's poisonous root, which is white, thick, and fleshy, with an unpleasant odor. The root may grow to an enormous size. It is said to grow to a length of two feet and become as thick as a man's arm, and occasionally growing to the size of a year-old child. This root, sometimes called Devil's turnip, has an interesting history. In the past, criminals would form it into the shape of a man and sell it as the mandrake root. These petty criminals would dig a hole around the root of a young plant and place a mold in the shape of a human figure for the root to grow into. The hole would be filled in, and the root would, in one summer, fill the mold. The criminal would then dig up the root and sell it as true mandrake.

Mandrake root was very valuable because it was thought to create love and fertility and bring good fortune and prosperity to an individual and to the household. Along with being an "imposter mandrake," white bryony may have been used as a man root in Europe long before the use of mandrake. A man root is a root that either grows in the shape of the human form or is carved into a little manikin or doll. This manikin, believed to have magical powers, is kept in a small coffin, often wrapped in fine cloth such as linen or silk. Certain rituals must be kept in order to maintain the power of the manikin, such as taking it out of its coffin a number of times during the year and bathing it. Other rituals involve giving it a token such as a small amount of money.

When maintained in this way, the manikin is supposed to give its owner wealth, love, and magical powers. It was thought to produce money for its owner and to assure his or her success in business. Persons who were wealthy without any visible source of income were thought to be in possession of a man root that created money.

Thus the traditional symbolism of the plant, with its root that was thought to bring financial security, is completely consistent with our homeopathic understanding of *Bryonia*. It is a remedy that represents the clinging aspect of the vine. Individuals needing this remedy are entangled with the material world in such a manner that they become obsessed with the need for money and security and lose the ability to enjoy other aspects of their lives. This one-sided view of life often leads to a kind of ossification and contraction, especially as a person ages. The fear of moving out into other realms of experience can then overtake the individual, and he or she become even more staid and conservative. It is no wonder that *Bryonia* is a remedy for arthritis and other aches and pains that are aggravated by motion.

RHUS TOXICODENDRON
POISON IVY

Rhus toxicodendron, poison ivy, was introduced into homeopathy by Hahnemann. The remedy is well known for its use in rheumatic conditions and injuries in which there is pain and stiffness that is aggravated by immobility or when the person begins to move. Continued movement improves the discomfort until fatigue sets in. Due to the effect of poison ivy on the skin, it is no surprise that poison ivy made into a homeopathic remedy would also address all kinds of skin eruptions. All symptoms treated by this remedy are better when the person is warm and worse in the cold. Because the symptoms treated are worse when the patient is still, those needing this remedy are very restless and physically uneasy.

Hahnemann noted the similarities and differences between *Rhus tox* and *Bryonia,* calling them two antagonistic sister remedies and used them both, alternately, to treat many of his patients during the typhus epidemic of 1813. These two remedies are also similar in that they are both made from clinging vines and those who benefit from them cling very strongly to the material world. Those needing *Rhus tox* are impatient to accomplish many things, particularly involving business. They worry about business or financial failure, and like people who require *Bryonia,* they dream of business and their business difficulties.

Along with worrying about business and finances, those who need *Rhus tox* are also anxious about their families. They have a lot of anxiety about their children and relatives. In general, the worry is obsessive, and they dream about the events of the day and even talk in their sleep about business difficulties. The mind, along with the body, cannot let go and rest, even in sleep. They become depressed and despondent because of constant apprehension that they cannot get out of their head. There seems to be no place for relaxation. They are restless and, at the same time stiff, with fixed ideas.

Out of touch with their inner life, the only expression of the inner state is through superstitious fears and anxieties. Their unconscious responds with dreams of their world collapsing, or they dream the world is on fire or coming to an end, an indication that they need to stop clinging and let go a bit or things will come tumbling down on them. These people have fears of killing their children, a fear that compensates for their overconcern. Given the paradoxical nature of the psyche, the opposite can be true as well, the overconcern for their children could be a compensation for the inner desire to be free from them.

In people who need *Rhus tox*, the connection with the rational world is well developed, and the world of the spirit remains in a younger, simpler state. This one-sided clinging to a rational view of the material world is compensated for through various fears of the existence of phenomenon that cannot be explained. These emerge from the unconscious as fears of being harmed by the unknown. These people have a fear of ghosts and become obsessed with the idea that there is some malicious and invisible being that appears to them at night. This can become so frightening that they attempt to escape its influence by getting out of bed and doing something else.

Suspicion and fear of being poisoned can become so bad that the patient may refuse to take the homeopathic remedy.

The above symptoms clarify how the clinging aspect of the vine relates to the poison ivy vine. This vine grows up a tree by putting out many little tendrils that cling voraciously to its host. Anyone who has ever tried to tear down these vines knows how difficult it is to remove them. Unfortunately, this voracious clinging in an individual creates a rigidity and stiffening of the mind and body that worsens as time goes on. *Rhus tox* is an important remedy in arthritis, when the body becomes more and more inflexible. The restlessness that is an attempt to relieve the stiffness becomes greater and infiltrates the mental state.

Fortunately, when this vine is given according to the law of similars, it can often help to relieve these symptoms and bring greater resilience into the mind and body.

PASSIFLORA INCARNATA
PASSIONFLOWER

Passiflora is a perennial twining vine with whitish flowers tinged with purple. The remedy is made from the leaf of the plant and was introduced into the homeopathic materia medica by the nineteenth-century homeopath Edwin M. Hale, M.D. Even though there are many reports of *Passiflora's* use by homeopathic physicians in the late nineteenth and early twentieth century, there has been no official proving of it as a remedy.

Passiflora has been used in small and large material doses for the treatment of insomnia, when the sleeplessness is caused by nervous sensitivity. *Passiflora* has also been used for treatment of neuralgia, trismus, chorea, and other spasmodic maladies. The symptoms are generally aggravated by mental worries, exhaustion, and mental excitement. The individual needing this remedy feels worse at night and after a meal but is better from remaining quiet. An important indication for *Passiflora* is that the tongue is clean.

There has been a history of some success in using *Passiflora* in the treatment of delirium tremens, alcoholism, and drug addiction. Dr. D. C. Buell successfully treated an old man with delirium tremens with teaspoonful doses of the plant. This not only cured his insomnia but also his craving for alcohol and morphine. Massimo Mangialavori mentions this remedy as useful for treatment of narcotic abuse.

Although *Passiflora* deserves a full proving, the clinical applications of this flowering vine indicate that it is a valuable remedy for alcohol and drug addiction. Its symbolic meaning is well known and, like the grapevine, is related to deep spiritual imagery.

Emanuel de Villegas, a Mexican Augustinian friar, first perceived the symbolism of the passionflower in 1650. According to Villegas, each part of the plant is related to an aspect of Christ's passion. The spiraling tendrils of the vine symbolize the lash of Christ's scourging, and the seventy-two radial filaments of the plant symbolize His crown of thorns. The top three stigmas represent the three nails that were placed into Christ's hands and feet and five lower anthers of the plant relate to Christ's five wounds. The red-purple stains on the flower indicate drops of Christ's blood.

Emanuel de Villegas's perception of the vine and its flower as a symbol of the passion of Christ has been accepted and passed on through the centuries. This association is so enduring that it is still held in the European and northern countries where the flower grows. The story is even known by indigenous people of the rain forest.

If we accept that alcoholism and drug addiction are spiritual diseases, then the spiritual symbolism surrounding *Passiflora,* along with its past history of use in treating those dependencies, indicate its value as a homeopathic remedy for substance abuse and addiction.

CLEMATIS ERECTA
VIRGIN'S BOWER

Clematis erecta was proved and introduced into the homeopathic materia medica by Hahnemann, and the full proving appears in his *Chronic Diseases.* This remedy is known for its action on the genitourinary system and particularly the testicles, and is an important remedy for orchitis. *Clematis erecta* has an effect on any glands that are very hard and swollen. *Clematis erecta* can also cause and therefore cure skin eruptions, many of which are very similar to the eruptions of *Rhus tox.*

The remedy is made from the leaf and stem of *Clematis erecta,* a flowering vine commonly known as virgin's bower. The common name is an allusion to the Virgin Mary, and in the Western language of flowers, *Clematis* symbolizes inner beauty. A member of the Rannunculae family, *Clematis* is related to *Pulsatilla.*

The clinging nature of this small vine is shown in the symptoms of homesickness and fear of being alone that may be cured by the remedy.

CHAPTER THIRTEEN

Milk Symbolism
First Food

Milk, as the first food for the infant, is a powerful symbol of the mother and of nurturing, of plenty and of fertility. Because of its association to the sublime and peaceful state of the suckling infant, and because of its innocent white quality, milk has always been a symbolic antidote against evil. In ancient Greece and Rome, milk was used in sacrifice to appease the gods of the underworld.

According to the *Ramayana,* the ancient narrative epic of India, churning the "Sea of Milk" produced the nectar of life. This created the nectar of immortality. An Ayurvedic text speaks of milk being mixed into "bliss bestowing soma" to become nectar of the gods.

Indeed, breast milk contains many opiate-like substances that produce the beatific state associated with both the peaceful breast-fed infant and the enlightened sage.

The breast itself, the chalicelike container that exudes warmth and comfort to the little one, continues to be a source of fascination, particularly to males, even into later life. In cases in which there has been early deprivation of mother and her nurturance, some people return to the drinking of soporific beverages and the taking of other mind-soothing substances, such as narcotics, in the attempt to create the peace and comfort of that early state of communion with the mother.

When researching the symbolism of milk, I had a dream in which a voice announced the following: "When the child is not nurtured by the parents, nature, in her bounty, brings forth a cow and the child is suckled by the great udder." This voice from the psyche was describing a psychological truth. When the actual parent does not nurture the child or abandons him or her, nature steps in and nurtures the child through the mother archetype. An animal mother such as a cow, as in my dream, often represents the mother archetype.[1]

> *Romulus and Remus were twin boys who were born to Rhea Silva, the daughter of a king. She had been forced by her uncle Amuilius to become a vestal virgin for political reasons, her vow of celibacy preventing her from bearing an heir. However, Mars, the god of war, visited her at the temple and she became pregnant. On hearing of the birth, Amuilius, who was afraid he might eventually be overthrown by the sons, ordered his servants to drown the twins. The servants, having compassion for the babes, placed them in a basket and tossed them into the Tiber River.*
>
> *They floated downstream until they landed near a sacred fig tree. There a woodpecker and a she-wolf discovered them, both sacred to the boys' father, Mars. They were suckled by the she-wolf and later raised by a friendly farmer and his wife.*

History has many such examples of children who have, for one reason or another, been left to the care of such foster parents, whether human or animal. Myths often describe heroes in their infancy as having been raised by an alternate mother. Moses was left in the bulrushes and later found and raised by the Pharaoh's daughter. Someone other than his own mother raised Hiawatha.

Alchemical literature contains many symbols of this phenomenon. One relevant to our subject is a woodcut of the earth as suckling mother. This illustration appears in Michael Maier's alchemical emblem book *Atalanta Fugiens*, which was first published in Latin in 1617 and contained the following epigram to accompany the woodcut:

His Nurse Is the Earth

Romulus is said to have been nursed at the coarse udders of a wolf,
But Jupiter to have been nursed by a goat, and these facts are said to be believed:
Should we then wonder if we assert
That the earth suckles the tender Child of the Philosophers with its milk?
If an insignificant animal nursed such great heroes,
Shall he not be great, who has the Terrestrial Globe as a nurse.[2]

Designated hero or not, many individuals brought up without proper nurturing must rely on a relationship to the mother archetype and are thus destined to the hero's journey in their lives. In this situation, the child has no intermediary to the archetype; therefore the child's path to individual wholeness is much more difficult.

When a mother and father provide healthy parenting, they substitute their personal presence for the ultimate archetypal experiences that may or may not come later in life. Without this early bonding, the individual must attempt to develop a relationship with the archetype within—a difficult feat that entails much suffering. Following this difficult path to individuation has many pitfalls, including those of depression, anxiety, and perhaps substance addiction. To make the inner connection and live in harmony with oneself and others without early childhood bonding to parents is indeed a hero's journey.

When the symptoms fit, an individual on such a journey can often be assisted in the quest for a healthy relationship to the great mother within through a homeopathic dilution of milk. The milk may be of a human mother, such as in *Lac humanum* or from other mammals. In his lectures on *Lac caninum,* or dog's milk, James Tyler Kent suggests the value of remedies made from the milk of various mammals:

> *All the milks should be potentized, they are our most excellent remedies, they are animal products and foods of early animal life and therefore correspond to the beginning of our innermost physical nature. If we had full provings of monkey's, cow's, mare's and human milk they would be of great value.*[3]

In Kent's time *Lac caninum, Lac felinum* (cat's milk), and *Lac vaccinum* (cow's milk) were proved by homeopathic physician Samuel Swan, M.D. Swan also proved some individual constituents of cow's milk, including *Lac defloratum* (skimmed milk), *Lac vaccinum coagulatum* (milk curds), and *Lac vaccinum flos* (cream from cow's milk). Koumiss, or fermented ass's milk, is mentioned in the old materia medicas, but no provings are mentioned. Since Kent's time, many more provings have been done on the milk of various mammals. In addition to the first remedies proved by Swan in the 1880s, the homeopathic materia medica now includes *Lac delphinum* (dolphin's milk), *Lac leoninum* (lion's milk), *Lac loxodonta Africana* (milk of the African elephant), *Lac lupinum* (wolf's milk), and *Lac equinum* (horse's milk)—all proven by Nancy Herrick. Also newly proven are *Lac caprinum* (goat's milk) and *Lac humanum* (human mother's milk).

Although the milks of different mammals have various unique qualities, they also have many similarities. Themes and symptoms shared by many of the milk remedies are as follows:

- Feelings of ugliness, with a feeling of revulsion for oneself and one's body
- Feelings of inferiority
- Delusions that one is separated from the world, isolated
- Dreams of being left behind by loved one's or relatives
- Dreams of snakes, fear of snakes
- Aversion or intolerance to milk
- Desire for salty food
- Aggravation before the menses
- Sore throat
- Constipation

Of these symptoms, the most frequently seen are the delusion of being separated from the world, dreams of being left behind by loved ones, and the dreams and fears of snakes. It is easy enough to understand the relationship of feeling alone and left behind by loved ones. It is a feeling that is often present in those who have not had the benefit of loving parenting in early childhood. The security that develops from the early bonding with the mother is not there or it has been damaged and turned into a need that can no longer be satisfied.

LAC CANINUM
BITCH'S MILK

Bitch's milk, which was proven by Swan in 1871, was well known in ancient medicine. The Greeks used it for erosion of the cervix and to expel the dead fetus. Great fear, apprehension accompanied by low self-esteem, and feelings of worthlessness are important indications for this remedy. Swan's provings of *Lac caninum* revealed an extraordinary number of dreams, fantasies, and fears about snakes. The fear of snakes is so prominent and extreme in this remedy that persons who need it can be frightened by simply glimpsing pictures of snakes in a magazine or watching a television show about the creatures. These people have very lively imaginations that are easily stimulated by the thought of any danger, but particularly concerning snakes.

The question arises, What is the symbolic significance of the snake in this remedy made from the milk of the dog? In order to understand the snake's significance, we must explore the relationship between the snake and what is represented by the milk itself—the mother. As in all remedies made from milk, the mother is an issue in *Lac caninum*. Persons needing it often have a history of difficulty with their mother that haunts them throughout their life.

The snake is a huge archetypal symbol that represents many energies, depending upon its context. The snake appears in different times and cultures as the symbol of the mother in her primal form. In Australian Aboriginal tales, she is the Rainbow Snake or great mother snake who emerges from deep inside of the earth to create the rivers and plants and animals. She is the beneficent creator, but she is also capable of punishing those who break her laws.

As has been previously mentioned, all archetypes have their polar opposites. Because of humanity's powerful association with the nurturing aspect of the mother archetype, it is often difficult to realize that the polar opposite of the archetype is the killing mother. The killing mother is she who is capable of destroying her child through violence, neglect, and withholding of her nurturance. This side is seen in spiritual symbols such as Kali, the Hindu goddess of destruction, and in the following story of Isis, where the snake represents the negative capacity of the mother archetype.

In *Symbols of Transformation*, Jung describes the psychological implications of the snake symbolism in regard to the mother, through an ancient Egyptian hymn. In the hymn, a poisonous snake created by his mother, Isis, bites the god Ra. This myth represents the polar energy of the mother, who kills and is also man's only security, as she is the source of life.

The hymn of the destruction of Ra not only shows the poisoning but continues to tell of the cure, which must be through that which caused the problem, the mother. Isis tells Ra that the only way he will be cleansed of the poison is to tell her his true name. In other words, she demands his essence or soul. Ra tells her his true name but is only partially cured and must return to his celestial abode on the back of the heavenly cow. Jung describes the significance of this symbolism:

> *The meaning of this symbolism becomes clear in the light of what we said earlier: the forward-striving libido which rules the conscious mind of the son demands separation from the mother, but his childish longing for her prevents this by setting up a psychic resistance that manifests itself in*

all kinds of neurotic fears–that is to say, in a general fear of life. The more a person shrinks from adapting himself to reality, the greater becomes the fear which increasingly besets his path at every point. Thus a vicious circle is formed: fear of life and people causes more shrinking back, and this in turn leads to infantilism and finally into the mother.[4]

In other words, the snake represents a morbid connection to the mother that cripples the individual with fear and apprehension. This is not the mother per se, but rather, the individual's connection with some part of the psychic energy of the mother figure that keeps him from letting go and growing out of this early stage of development. The real source is in the unconscious. The snake represents a debilitating fear of the instinctive inner self that is projected out into the world. This fear prevents him from action. The world becomes a terrifying place, in which anything may happen and any decision may have terrible consequences. This causes the well-known wavering symptoms seen in the *Lac caninum* patient. Neither the mind nor the body can decide which direction to turn, leading to changeable symptoms that move from one side to the other and then back again and a type of indecisiveness that almost exactly parallels the psychic state.

The patient can become paralyzed with fear, beginning to doubt his or her own mind and developing an obsession with avoiding change. Added to this fear is an overly lively imagination that imagines the worst and leads to many anticipatory fears.

Lac caninum is well known as a remedy for premenstrual syndrome, particularly for swelling of the breasts before menses. This is particularly disturbing for the woman needing this remedy, as she often has great sensitivity about her body and especially her weight. She considers herself, and especially her body, ugly beyond repair, "feeling that she was loathsome, horrible, mass of disease" as one prover reported. This distorted body image can easily lead to an eating disorder or compulsive dieting.

Those who need *Lac caninum* have the sense of living on the edge; a very thin edge with an underlying nameless terror. This terror can be compared with living on the edge of a snake pit. The mother has become internalized as the negative mother archetype in the form of the snake. This terrible creature coils herself around the psyche, leaving the individual in a constant state of anxiety. That which should have been nourishing milk has been transformed into a source of venomous psychic energy that continues to poison the individual even in adult life.

The state requiring *Lac caninum,* in its very early stages, can be seen in the dynamics between a nursing mother and a child. Often, both mother and child experience more than the healthy ambivalence about weaning at an appropriate age. This can happen even after the child has developed teeth and is eating solid food. The child flies into a fit of rage at any attempt on the part of the mother to wean or separate from it. The mother, in her attempt to do her best for the child, becomes its unwilling slave.

In these cases, the nursing mother needing *Lac caninum* may have never resolved her own early connection with her mother and is now, during breast-feeding, experiencing the return of many early emotions.

She wants to move on with her life and yet she wants to remain in the "participation mystique," or merging with her child and her own inner mother. She wants to remain with the child for reasons beyond the actual needs of the child. This inner conflict and indecision, between the desire to stay a suckling infant and the desire to be an adult, is typical of people who need *Lac caninum* and other milk remedies.

Lac caninum, well known for drying up the milk of nursing mothers, can help both the child and the mother move on to another stage of development in their relationship. Given to the nursing mother, it will help both the child and the mother lessen their fears and move away from the coils of the crippling "snake mother" and into a greater sense of autonomy.

For those who are not so fortunate to receive this remedy when needed at an early age, the path to developing some degree of autonomy can be more difficult and prolonged. Their wavering and dependent natures require much attention and patience on the part of the homeopath, who may be required to answer many phone calls and help these patients through difficult times before they are able to stand on their own.

Lac caninum can, with time—and often with the help of *Lyssin* as a complementary remedy—assist an individual in lessening many of his or her fears and aid in the development of a sense of self. The remedy helps in this process just as, at the end of the Egyptian hymn, Ra, still wounded, is carried home on the back of the heavenly cow.

LAC FELINUM
CAT'S MILK

Lac felinum, or cat's milk, was introduced into the homeopathic materia medica by Swan. It is known for eye symptoms and, especially, shooting pains in the eye. Nervous trembling of the hands and fear of sharp pointed objects, a fear of falling downstairs and extreme conscientiousness are also indicators that *Lac felinum* might be needed. Since 1995, several homeopaths have done clinical investigations of this remedy, including a synthetic remedy picture based on an observation of eleven patients by Karl-Josef Mueller and Gerhard Ruster.[5] According to Marie-Louise von Franz, in her book *The Cat: A Tale of Feminine Redemption*,[6] the cat has been an archetypal symbol since ancient Egypt. The Egyptians considered cats to be sacred animals, and Bastet, the cat goddess, was the daughter of the goddess Isis. Celebrations in honor of Bastet were fun-filled, bawdy festivals, full of music and lascivious allusions to sex. People rode down the Nile on barges, and women lifted their skirts and showed their bare bottoms, "mooning" the cheering audiences on the shore. Because the cat goddess was associated with fertility, there were sexual orgies that were believed to increase the fertility of the people, their animals, and the land.

The cat goddess was also associated with music, and cats were often shown with the musical instrument of Isis, the sistrum, which is similar to a tambourine. In all, the cat was a very positive symbol, connected with fertility, music, bawdy celebration, and sensual pleasure. Although, as with all symbols, the cat had a dark side and was associated with the land of the dead, it was the light and pleasurable side of the cat that was emphasized at this time.

It wasn't until the Middle Ages that the cat became a symbol of evil and the power of the devil. The cat was often seen accompanying a witch, and some women were said to put the power of their souls into a black cat. This belief probably had much to do with the Catholic church and its disassociation from the instincts, sexuality, and feminine power. The devilish aspect of the cat, according to von Franz, has only been emphasized since the time of Christianity and has to do with the patriarchal banishing of the feminine shadow. Similar to witches, cats were persecuted, and there were terrible cat hangings. All of this was thought to get rid of evil influences. The bawdy, joyous, and irreverent side of the feminine energy, so enjoyed in ancient times, could not be tolerated by the church and slipped into the darkness where, projected onto women who delved into their own power and onto the independent cat, feminine energy became the object of fear and hatred.

Although the cat allows us to be near it, this association is always on the cat's terms. Unlike the dog, which becomes greatly attached to its master, the cat always maintains its independence. The cat likes to come and go as it pleases and may even secretly maintain more than one home, allowing itself to be fed and pampered by more than one family.

The cat is a symbol of independence and often shows up in dreams when there is a need for compensation for an overly dependent life with too little freedom. Marie-Louise von Franz describes her interpretation of the cat in the dreams of a certain type of woman:

> You often see cat dreams in women who have no independence, who are too doggishly attached to their husband and children, and then, I always stress what a cat does. A cat goes its own way. It knows what it wants and goes its own way. A cat comes for certain feeding times, and then it's really friendly. But when it wants to leave, "Meeow," you have to let it out. It's very cruel to imprison a cat. You can keep a dog in a flat but to keep a cat inside a flat and never let it out is really cruel, because it needs the independence; it needs its own life.[7]

Here we have the cat as a symbol of the need for independence; the need for a woman to be able, like to cat, to go her own way. On a collective level, the change in the way the cat has been viewed shows the change in societal acceptance of feminine power. The early celebration of feminine sensuality and independence moved to a level of disassociation that lead to delegating these lusty feminine energies into the collective shadow, where it was feared and hated. Unfortunately, due to the continued prominence of patriarchy, much of the negative view of the feminine persists to this day; this contin-ued delegation of feminine power to the shadow makes it very difficult for both men and women to realize their feminine nature. When the need to free the feminine nature from the bonds of restriction is of primary impor-tance in an individual's life, *Lac felinum* may be an appropriate remedy. In the overview of eleven patients who responded favorably to the remedy, Mueller and Ruster found "the desire for liberty, the wish to be a free agent, to be one of the most frequently occurring desires in *Lac felinum*." The provers also had a strong aversion to doing anything against their will and a desire to preserve their independence in relationship.

In an article in the international homeopathic journal *Homeopathic Links*, Alize Timmerman, a homeopathic practitioner and teacher from the Netherlands, writes about the remedy *Lac felinum*. The article, "The Symbol in a Remedy as a Key Factor," explains the antagonism between being dependent and childlike and the need to be independent, through the case of a young woman who was successfully treated with *Lac felinum*.[8]

Anne Wirtz, a Dutch homeopath who had successfully treated fifteen people with *Lac felinum,* only one of whom was male, has similar findings. In an article in the same issue of *Homeopathic Links,* she describes the basic pattern of the person requiring *Lac felinum* as a woman who felt abused and neglected reacting by becoming rebellious and independent, creating an "I don't need anybody" attitude.[9]

Although one shouldn't immediately connect the behavior of the actual cat with the remedy, we can see from clinical experience that there is a theme of the need for independence in *Lac felinum.* The symbolism attached to the cat over centuries reinforces this theme, especially in reference to the changing attitudes toward the feminine.

LAC DEFLORATUM
SKIMMED COW'S MILK

Lac defloratum, or skimmed cow's milk, was potentized and proved by Swan along with two other cow's milk remedies, *Lac vaccinum* (whole milk), and *Lac vaccinum* flos (cream). *Lac defloratum* is a major remedy for milk allergy or lactose intolerance, and for diabetes. When a patient has migraine headaches and an allergy to milk ,or headaches with profuse urination, we must consider *Lac defloratum.* Given the frequency of milk allergies, and the well-developed mental state in Swan's proving, it is surprising that skimmed cow's milk is not used more frequently in homeopathic practice.

The cow has been domesticated for thousands of years, and humans have consumed cow milk more than the milk of any other species. In the past, even the smallest farmstead had at least one cow whose milk—and the meat from her offspring—provided a major source of food. The leather from her hide provided clothing and sometimes even shelter. Therefore, the cow was endowed with rich symbolic significance.

Throughout history, and in varied civilizations, the cow has been a symbol of Mother Earth as giver of wealth, fertility, and plenty. Hathor, the ancient Egyptian cow goddess, represented fertility, wealth, rebirth, and the heavenly mother of the sun. She was ruler of the body of the sky, the living soul of trees, the smiling goddess of joy, music, and dance. An amulet representing Hathor was often worn by early Egyptian women to assure their fertility.

Hathor was called the great celestial cow, who created the world and all that it contains, including the sun. She was represented as a cow-headed goddess or as a cow, her sacred animal. As protector of women, Hathor was supposed to preside at their toilet. She was goddess of joy and love, music and song.

Nourishing the living with her milk, Hathor is represented in the form of a cow, suckling the Pharaoh. She was even more nurturing toward the dead, welcoming them on their arrival in the other world. She would carry those who knew how to call upon her into the underworld.[10] According to *The Penguin Dictionary of Symbols*, the cow Ahat (another name for the cow-goddess) was the origin of all manifestations and mother of the sun. The Ahat amulet depicting the head of the sacred cow with a solar disk between its horns was used to transmit "warmth" into mummified bodies. This custom arose from the belief that when the sun, Ra, dropped for the first time below the horizon, the cow goddess sent fiery beings to succor him until morning so that he did not lose his heat.[11]

The cow, once revered as the source of all nourishment, connected with Mother Earth, is now one of the most used and abused of all animals on the planet. Just as we abuse the cow, we abuse Mother Earth. We have lost our mythological connection with the cow, and with the earth. We human beings have fallen to the point that we abuse that which sustains us.

Once the symbol of riches and fertility, the cow has become a manufactured animal, bred and pumped full of hormones and antibiotics so she will provide huge amounts of milk. Her calves are quickly fattened with food that often contains parts of their sisters and brothers. They are slaughtered without any compassion, to be wrapped in plastic and consumed without any thought that the meat was once a living being. Is it any wonder that we now have mad cow disease? The theme of abuse and violence toward someone who nourishes and cares for others is seen in the short dream proving done by Rajan Sankaran. The provers had dreams of animals being tied and beaten, of being neglected, and of an obese, elderly woman being beaten mercilessly. Sankaran lists a theme of seeing others of his group being beaten and abused by other people or authorities, but being helpless against it.

This abuse toward the cow, the symbol of Mother Earth, implies a disconnection from all that is nurturing and caring, and the ensuing loneliness. We see symptoms associated with this disconnection and loneliness from Swan's original proving in Allen's *Nosodes:*

> *Does not want to see or talk to anyone. Doesn't care to live; question as to quietest and most certain way of hastening one's death. Imagines that all her friends will die and that she must go to a convent. Dreams of going on a journey, and was separated from party, and had to walk a long distance, and arrive at station just in time to see train start off.*

The main theme is of being abandoned or forsaken, being neglected by friends and community. This feeling, along with symbolic connections to abuse and violence toward caregivers, indicates the value of *Lac defloratum* for persons who have been victimized. These people are most often mild and sweet-natured and have an allergy to milk.

However, allergy to milk may be also connected with the way the cow is raised. Commercial milk and dairy products from abused animals pumped full of antibiotics and growth hormones are most likely an obstacle to cure and should not be consumed by those wishing to improve or maintain their health.

MIND AND DREAM SYMPTOMS OF THE MILK REMEDIES

Remedy	Mind	Dreams
Lac vaccinum flos (Cream from cow's milk)		Horrible dreams. Saw a dead person in a coffin.
Lac defloratum (Skimmed cow's milk)	Fear of narrow places. Depression, doesn't care to live, what is the quietest and most certain way to die. Imagines all her friends will die and she must go to a convent. Vacillation Feeling poisoned	Dreamed a large snake was in bed. He had to go on a journey and was separated from party and had to walk a long distance arriving at station just in time to see the train start off.
Lac vaccinum (Cow's milk)		Dreams of trying to lay out a corpse.
Lac caninum (Bitch's milk)	Thinks she is looked down upon by everyone, that she is of no importance. Imagines she wears someone else's nose, she is dirty. Fear of snakes. Attacks of rage and cursing.	Dreamed a large snake was in bed. Of urination, traveling, missing trains, etc. She was one mass of sores with worms.
Lac caprinum (Goat's milk)	Shameless sexuality. Fear he will lose his high position because he has something sexual to hide. (Falling from a pedestal.) Fear of being attacked.	
Lac delphinum (Dolphin's milk)	Frightened but calm. Feeling of separation from others. Desire to be connected. Laughter and play. Exertion, swimming.	Swing two girls around playfully. During a trip wife packed to leave and go off with other people. Dreams of children.
Lac equinum (Mare's milk)	Irritable and impatient, makes mistakes. Confrontation. Frustration.	Violent dreams, people being shot, aliens, fighting, killing.
Lac leoninum (Lion's milk)		Dreams of snakes.
Lac loxodonta Africana (African elephant's milk)	Delusions, floating in air.	Dreams, violent, murder. Poverty, disease. Not enough food. Hungry. Homeless.
Lac humanum (Human mother's milk)	Detached, aversion to company, indifference to everything, to the suffering of others. Isolation. Independence/dependence. Feeling of two wills.	Dreams of babies, family, buildings. Left alone in the world. Aunt throws her off the train. Surrounded by snakes.
Lac felinum (Cat's milk)	Morbid consciousness, every fault seems a serious crime. Fear of falling downstairs. Fear of pointy things. Feels dirty. Dependency/independence.	Sexual dreams. Dreams of being pursued for rape. Earthquakes.
Lac lupinum (Wolf's milk)	Feels comfortable with risk, with danger. Does not care for what others think. Indifferent, sits and observes the world going by.	Of bears, animals, or cars. Of being safe in a dangerous situation, danger.

CHAPTER FOURTEEN

The Seven Metals of the Alchemists

The concept of the microcosm within the macrocosm is an attempt to understand how a human being relates to the entire universe and the interrelatedness of all things in the universe. It is an idea that has been explored by philosophers, healers, and writers throughout millennia and is a question that has been investigated by the alchemists using the doctrine of the seven metals. In times when a dominant religion prevailed, these doctrines belonged primarily to the church, and any dispute was considered heresy.

Since the Enlightenment, the question of how human beings relate to the universe has been delegated to the world of science and rational thought. Even though the new physics shows us that the defined boundaries that we once thought separated all matter do not exist, human consciousness has not yet been able to integrate these findings into daily life. Most current science, and particularly medicine, views life from an extremely materialistic perspective, breaking down the world into individual pieces, each to be examined and treated as isolated entities. Human beings are viewed as an accumulation of separate parts that can be treated separately, and in some cases, may be disposed of and replaced with other parts. In the current atmosphere of rational and materialistic thinking, it is generally unacceptable to speak of the interconnectedness of all of the body parts, never mind the interconnectedness of human beings and the universe.

Systems such as the seven metals of the alchemists were an attempt to explain the connection between humanity and the universe in symbolic form. Because this type of symbolic thinking does not fit into our present and dominant worldview, it is considered primitive and outdated. However, even though this belief belongs to an earlier age, it represents wisdom that we would do well to investigate, as it may lead to a synergistic blend of symbolic wisdom and rational thinking that could be closer to the most recent and expansive discoveries of modern science.

Because of the scientific process of provings combined with information from clinical experience and toxicology, homeopaths are in an excellent position to explore the relationship between matter and the human mind and body. With the addition of knowledge of wisdom from the ancients, such as the seven metals, it is also possible to explore the interaction between a particular substance, the body/mind, and the rest of the universe.

The alchemists believed that the heavens and the earth and the inner and outer worlds were linked; what was in the heaven and in the stars was in the earth. This was a linking of matter and spirit, a linking of the earth and the realm of the gods. According to such correspondences, the alchemists designated seven metals in the earth that were associated with the seven most visible planets. In many myths and legends from various cultures, as well as in alchemy, the seven metals and their planets were arranged in the following hierarchy, beginning with lead and ending with gold.

Lead = Saturn
Tin = Jupiter
Iron = Mars
Copper = Venus
Mercury = Mercury
Silver = Moon
Gold = Sun

Because the metals connected the microcosm of the human body with the macrocosm, alchemists, such as Paracelsus, used the concept of the seven metals in their medicine. According to the alchemists, each metal represented particular organs, tissues, and bodily systems and corresponded to a day of the week and times of the day, much like the Chinese model of the Five Elements. Particular healing herbs were said to belong to one of the metals and were influenced by its corresponding planet. These, in turn, could treat imbalances of the body, mind, and spirit that belonged to that planet. For example, copper was associated with the planet Venus, the goddess of love, and the emotion of love. These corresponded to the generative organs, and problems in these areas were treated with copper and with herbs such as foxglove, marshmallow, and mugwort, which corresponded to Venus.

Unlike the Five Elements concept of the Chinese, where the elements were cyclical and nonhierarchical, the alchemists viewed the seven metals as a process of evolution. This process, they said, might need to be repeated many times, but eventually it would end with the final step, that of transformation into gold.

Alchemy and the process of transformation of lead into gold can be viewed from three different perspectives. The first is the materialistic perspective. This views the alchemical opus as a physical process, an early form of chemistry that is concerned with physical work in the laboratory. The second is to see the alchemists' quest as an attempt to transform a substance into a medicine, and the third is to understand their work as the transformation of the alchemist. Here the process of transformation of a substance is seen as a projection of the psyche of the alchemist. This is the realm of soul alchemy or inner alchemy—the task of the inner transmutation of forces within the soul. Here the philosopher's stone (the goal of the work, or as it is referred to in alchemy, the opus) is a state in which various parts of the soul are integrated. Jung explored the relationship between alchemy and individuation from this perspective. Although all three perspectives are needed to understand alchemy, the second and third views are especially relevant to the field of homeopathy.

Hahnemann knew about alchemy and mentions some of the alchemists in his work. He was especially interested in metals and said that he doubted that any metal was "destitute of curative powers."[1] The seven metals have been used in homeopathy for over 150 years and play an important role in our materia medica. Hahnemann himself proved six of them, the exception being *Plumbum*. Although proven around 1880, thirty-seven years after his death, Hahnemann used *Plumbum* in his practice, though he never proved it.

The hierarchy of the seven metals symbolize a process of development; the transformation of lead into gold. From the provings and clinical information on the use of the seven metals as homeopathic remedies, we can see a theme that is parallel to the alchemists' view of these elements. In the lead, or *Plumbum*, state, human consciousness is confronted with a very basic truth, that all life processes contain death. When this is accepted and integrated into the psyche, one moves on to the challenges brought forth by tin, or *Stannum*. These challenges are centered on the need to be inspired and expanded into a lively state that will allow for further progress. Iron, or *Ferrum*, then brings forth the test of dealing with one's warrior energy in a balanced way, for the path of development requires courage and the ability to set boundaries. Only then does copper, or *Cuprum*, offer the opportunity for the experience of love and beauty to flow and be enjoyed.

Mercury, or Mercurius, the fleet-footed messenger who moves between heaven, Earth and the underworld, must be dealt with in order to move toward the noble metals of silver and gold. *Mercurius* confronts us with the need for communication on levels that are previously considered to be impossible or absurd and opens the gate to hell as well as heaven. In this stage, Mercurius, ever the trickster, makes one acutely aware of the living reality of the pairs of opposites.

After opening the gate to the opposites, the integration of the female, lunar energies are stimulated by the noble silver, or *Argentum*. Here the adept must learn the value of the passive forces and the deep unconscious before finally reaching the aim of the opus—gold, or *Aurum*. The test of gold is perhaps the most dangerous, as it necessitates a breaking down of the ego, a process that is most often associated with death and dying. But if this test of gold is met, there is a powerful inner transformation. From the perspective of soul alchemy, this is the transformation of lead into gold.

The alchemists wrote of the need to continually "wash" the metals through a process that required blackness, or nigredo, and then a whitening phase, or albedo. The nigredo not only refers to the process of heating and blackening the substance but also, from the perspective of inner alchemy, to the need to move into the dark or shadowy parts of the psyche and integrate those energies. This process purifies the shadow energies and eventually causes the cleansing or whitening phase. It is also written that this process needs to continue many times. Some texts say seven times for each metal; others write of the need for countless times.

Through this process, each metal, in both its earthly as well as its heavenly qualities, was thought to become transformed and transmuted into the next higher level, until the goal of the opus, the transformation of lead into gold, was accomplished. This can be understood from a psychological perspective to mean that there are archetypal configurations within the human psyche with which the ego identifies. Inner transformation or inner alchemy requires that the ego differentiate the godlike archetypal aspect of the metal from the earthbound aspect of it. If the ego identifies with the archetypal aspect of the metal, the heavenly planet with its associate god, the ego becomes inflated. On the other hand, if functioning unconsciously, the archetypal energy of the metal may take possession of the ego.

What is necessary is to become conscious of the relationship between the heavenly aspect and the earthly aspect, that is, to transform the metals alchemically so that the parts become refined and transformed into a substance that can be used in a way that helps to transform the individual and gives the gods their due by actualizing them in the individual ego.

Thus, the path of individuation may be compared with the transmutation of the base underworld metal to the more heavenly aspect; sublimation of the psychic energy of basic desires and carnal appetites transforms them to a higher level and reintegrates them into a more balanced existence.

Although the alchemists used the hierarchy of metals as general stages to guide them in diagnosis and treatment of disease, from the perspective of homeopathic therapy a particular metal is needed only when the individual exhibits physical, general, and emotional symptoms found in the provings or known clinical application of the particular metal. Given those guidelines, the alchemical significance of the metal, with its corresponding planet and hierarchy, may enhance our understanding of the underlying processes indicated in the homeopathic materia medica. It may also help us to relate more intimately to the remedy and open our hearts and minds to the connection between the macrocosm and the microcosm.

Although the following materia medica will concentrate on the seven metals themselves, understanding the metals may possibly extend to an understanding of salts of the seven metals or of plants that contain a large amount of the metal. Where multiple factors are present along with the basic themes of the metals, we may need to investigate a salt or a plant that contains that metal along with other components.

PLUMBUM METALLICUM
LEAD

Saturn—The Grim Reaper

"Death is a integral part of life"

Plumbum was proved by Hartlaub, Trinks, Hering and Nenning around 1880. The full proving and symptoms from cases of lead poisoning appear in Allen's *Encyclopedia of Pure Materia Medica*. The proving shows a complex mental state that includes delirium, apathy, fear of being attacked or assassinated, and mental deterioration. On the physical level there is constricting, cramping, and neuralgic pains, as well as paralysis and convulsions. Those who may benefit from the remedy are extremely chilly, with emaciation and numbness of the limbs.

Symptoms of lead poisoning include weight loss, anemia, apathy, and loss of recently acquired developmental skills in children. Many gastrointestinal symptoms, including cramping, constricting, and radiating pains, are also associated. Chronic lead poisoning can lead to localized neuritis and paralysis of the related muscles, as well as causing sclerotic lesions in the central nervous system. According to John Henry Clarke, M.D., English homeopath and author of *A Dictionary of Practical Materia Medica,* the best-known symptoms among painters and lead manufacturers exposed to lead are colic and wrist drop.

When the early alchemists referred to lead, they were referring to more than the actual physical lead, but rather lead as Saturn. Their understanding of this basic substance in the alchemical process can be understood through a legend from Egyptian alchemy.

In the legend, Set, the god of darkness, killed Osiris by making a leaden coffin and inviting many people, including Osiris to a party. There, Set served much wine and invited the drunken guests to enter the coffin to see who would fit. When Osiris got into the coffin, Set put on the lid, covered it with lead, and threw the coffin into the sea, where the divine god lay, suffocated by the lead.

This phenomenon of spirit deeply imprisoned in matter, where nothing is allowed to escape into the outside world, is what the alchemists are referring to when they speak of lead. One way of looking at their quest is as an attempt to free the limited aspects of themselves and move to a more universal sphere; to release the divine embedded within the dense matter of lead.

These ancient chemists knew the poisonous nature of lead, and it is not unreasonable to imagine that more than one alchemist was poisoned while attempting an alchemical experiment on this substance. Because of its poisonous qualities, the alchemists associated lead with Saturn, the god of limitation and death. Lead as Saturn was portrayed as the Grim Reaper, a skeleton sharpening his scythe, and was thought to be responsible for moving individuals through the trials and necessary separations that mark out every life cycle.

Saturn cuts the cord of the newborn infant and pushes the elderly to accept that they are no longer in the bloom of youth. Lead as Saturn represents the necessary death of the old state in order to move to the next stage of development. The infant must die in order for the child to be created; old cells must die to make room for a renewed vitality in the body. Without this death process, the human body and psyche would stagnate, become toxic, and die. The refusal of the ego to accept this death process or the body's inability to cleanse itself through death and renewal is the state of *Plumbum.*

When lead, as the Saturn aspect of an individual, is out of balance, the individual refuses to give up attachments. This state entombs one in a particular stage of development. This entombment may be seen on the physical level as retardation of bone formation, or it may occur in the thinking process as slowness of speech and inability to comprehend. On the emotional level it may be experienced as a refusal to give up emotional states that are no longer appropriate to a particular age, such as childish behavior in an adult.

The homeopathic remedy *Plumbum* is well known as a remedy for slowly developing diseases of the nervous and circulatory system. It is used for arteriosclerosis in persons who have lived a one-sided, materialistic existence. If the history of the case is examined, we see that the thought processes had become sclerotic long before the appearance of the circulatory problems. Here the thinking process has been limited to a very one-sided way of looking at life, in which the individual is limited to a very small aspect of the human capacity for thought.

The individual needing *Plumbum* refuses to accept the natural evolution of life and insists on keeping things the way that they feel they should be. This can lead to either a state of detachment, melancholy, and coldness, or into a state of intense jealousy, ambition, and hysteria. Either way, a supreme effort is made to try to cheat Saturn out of his natural processes. In his *Lectures on Materia Medica*, James Tyler Kent describes the hysterical aspect of *Plumbum* and the "cheating" aspect:

> Plumbum *produces an inclination to deceive, to cheat. The Acetate of lead produced in a woman, who took a little of it for suicide, a confirmed hysterical state. She would be in a hysterical condition for hours when anyone was looking at her. When she thought no one was near she would get up, walk about, look in the glass to see how handsome she was, but when she heard a foot on the steps she would lie on the bed and appear to be unconscious. She would bear much pricking and you could scarcely tell she was breathing.* Plumbum *establishes a hysterical state in the economy; an inclination to deceive, to feign sickness; to exaggerate one's ills; and it goes to the root of the evil providing the symptoms agree.*[2]

Kent does not describe the "root of evil" behind the deception and cheating found within the *Plumbum* state. However, in many cases, the reason behind the hysteria and cheating is an unwillingness to let go of a one stage and "die" into a new state of maturity.

Eventually, the debilitating and death-producing aspect of Saturn wins out, in spite of, or perhaps assisted by, the unwillingness of the organism to move forward into the necessary death inherent within psychic and bodily development. There is a gradual paralysis of the organs and the nerves of the body. The nerves and muscles slow down their activity, and the whole system becomes sluggish. The mind becomes slow and unable to think, comprehension becomes difficult. The whole system becomes leaden and heavy.

Eventually, the body begins to waste away, and the patient becomes the picture of the Grim Reaper himself, nothing but a skeleton.

Another symptom complex that is found in the provings of *Plumbum* is the fear of assassination. We can easily understand this fear in light of the denial of the necessary Saturnian movement in life. In the *Plumbum* state, the ego fights very hard to keep the life experience at a desired level, but Saturn is more powerful and continually pushes the individual toward death. In other words, the Grim Reaper's pushing toward the necessary dying processes inherent in human evolution is resisted and felt as the imminent possibility of assassination.

Plumbum is an important remedy for post-polio syndrome, a situation in which, many years after recovery from polio, an individual begins to have increased weakness, neuropathy, and other symptoms of breakdown of motor neurons. It has been shown that 80 percent of these individuals are extremely hardworking, perfectionists; super achievers who have learned to deny their bodily feelings and deny their disabilities. According to Dr. Richard Bruno, recognized as the world's foremost expert on post-polio sequelae, a majority of patients with PPS exhibit Type A behavior and are unable to express emotion or admit to having pain. Their anxiety and fear of criticism create a pattern where they tend to work until their physical symptoms prevent them from continuing. Only upon becoming totally exhausted do they rest until they can again push themselves to work until their symptoms force them to rest once more. In light of our discussion, they can be seen as denying the Saturnian process of death of motor neurons and pushing through. This strategy does not work and leads to greater weakness and debility.

When the symptoms fit, homeopathic doses of lead can help individuals toward realization and connection with their body and help them to take the rest that is so essential in relieving many of the symptoms of this syndrome.

Plumbum is most commonly used in cases of neurological diseases and paralysis, but these diseases exist in the organism long before the physical symptoms become obvious. If we are able to recognize the *Plumbum* state in its seed form, through understanding the mental state that precedes the physical, we may be able to help individuals who need this remedy to accept the god of death. In accepting Saturn, those needing the homeopathic remedy *Plumbum* can be helped to live a healthier and fuller life.

STANNUM METALLICUM
TIN

Jupiter–Joy, Laughter, and Expansion
"A flash of inspiration empowers and enlivens the soul."

Samuel Hahnemann, who prepared *Stannum metallicum* from the "finest leaf" of tin, first introduced the remedy into the homeopathic materia medica. *Stannum* is known for weakness, especially in the chest, and for symptoms that gradually increase and decrease throughout the day. People who need *Stannum* are sad and weepy, which aggravates the symptoms. *Stannum* is a tubercular remedy; it is recommended for people whose lungs are very weak, with a feeling of emptiness in the chest and problems with the voice because of weakness.

Tin in its pure state is rarely toxic because it cannot be readily absorbed by the body and is easily eliminated. When tin occurs as a salt or in compounds, however, it can be highly toxic, causing paralysis and neurological damage. It also affects the eyes, skin, and respiratory system and, as stannous chloride, can cause damage to the DNA.

One stage up from *Plumbum,* tin was the second metal in the alchemists' hierarchy of metals. *Stannum* was associated with the planet Jupiter and the god Zeus or Jove, who is connected with joy and laughter and expansion. The word *jovial* is derived from his name. Zeus's thunderbolt, with its zigzag shape, is the Arabic character for Jupiter, and the Greek initial for Zeus and tin was associated with this thunderbolt. Some say that tin imitates the voice of Zeus's thunderbolt, with the bright and crackling "cry" it emits when it is bent.

Zeus's weapon, the thunderbolt or lightning, is the symbol of intuition and spiritual enlightenment or a sudden flash of inspiration. It is a sign of power and strength capable of restoring equilibrium and vigor. As with all symbols, the thunderbolt has two sides; it has the ability to destroy as well as enlighten.

The ability of lightning to inspire as well as destroy is shown in a ritual from the Andean highlands of Peru. Only the most senior shamans who wish to gain abilities from this powerful force of nature climb to the highest snow-covered peaks of the Andes and call on the forces of nature to bring forth the lightning. When struck by the lightning, the shamans either receive great power and abilities or are killed.

Lightning is a powerful symbol in many societies, representing the virility of the creator. Lightning was also a symbol used by Paracelsus and the alchemists, to whom it indicated the liberating flash of unexpected and overpowering inspiration, resulting in a change of the psychic condition.

In contrast to the qualities of joy, energy, virility, and inspiration associated with the symbolic nature of tin, the homeopathic remedy *Stannum* is known for symptoms of weakness, depletion, and inability for deep inspiration because of weakness of the lungs. What is less known about the remedy is that the provings also show many symptoms related to the expansive, jovial state typical of Zeus. According to the *Millennium Repertory,* these symptoms include exuberance, ecstasy, mischievousness, and cheerfulness, as well as benevolence and sociability. Moreover, like the lustful Zeus, symptoms of lasciviousness, passion, and an amorous disposition show up.

In his *Encyclopedia of Pure Materia Medica,* Allen writes that those needing *Stannum* are excited and inclined to storms of anger. Also, remarkably, these people could be joyful, talkative, and sociable.[3]

The expansive healthy and inspired state of *Stannum* shows us the influence of Jupiter and Zeus. The other side of the coin is the weakness and lack of inspiration in the body and the mind. People report despair from exhaustion, weakness of memory, and indecision. These people persist in nothing, have an aversion to mental work, and cry all the time, but the crying makes them feel worse. These *Stannum* patients are so weak that they want to be alone because they don't have the energy to be with others and speak to them. They cannot get any work done and fritter away their time. There is a feeling of emptiness in the chest. A *Stannum* patient will point to his or her chest and say, "I feel emptiness inside of me." Or they will complain that the weakness is located in their chest. These individuals are so weak that they can barely speak. They often have weakness of the larynx and loss of voice because of mucus in the larynx.

Stannum is an important remedy in chronic fatigue, asthma, and other lung conditions with sadness and weeping. The physical conditions of *Stannum* are often long-standing, and there may have been a history of tuberculosis, asthma, or other lung conditions. The weakness can come on after overwork, financial loss, or another reversal of fortune. The unconscious compensates for the inability to get anything done with dreams of splendor and greatness. There are also dreams of explosions and fires, symbolizing the energy and heat that is missing in waking life.

The weakness, lack of motivation, and difficulty breathing point to the great need for power, strength, and inspiration as symbolized by Zeus's thunderbolt, the signature of tin. In its homeopathic dilution, tin, like the thunderbolt has the ability to enliven and enlighten the individual. *Stannum* helps the patient move to a new level of physical vitality and alleviate sadness, thus allowing the Jovial qualities of joy, laughter, and expansion to flourish.

FERRUM METALLICUM
IRON

Mars—Fire, War and Battle
"Winning the battle of opposing forces is an inside job."

Hahnemann prepared *Ferrum metallicum* from triturated iron filings and introduced it into the homeopathic materia medica. Much of his knowledge was from proving the substance, but a great deal of the information on this remedy was drawn from symptoms caused by the drinking of water with high iron content. Iron is an important trace mineral in the body and is especially important in the formation of hemoglobin, but in larger doses, it is toxic and can cause anemia. Other symptoms of iron poisoning include liver and kidney failure and cardiovascular collapse.

As a homeopathic remedy, iron is known as a treatment for anemia, especially when it occurs after hemorrhage in weak, pale persons who flush easily. The typical *Ferrum* patient is chilly, often obese, with irregular and changeable moods, and is ameliorated by slow motion.

The alchemists considered Mars, in the form of iron, to be a preservative against evil influences. For Paracelsus, iron corresponded to the body that has been purified by fire.

As the god of battle, Mars was also a diabolical instrument of war and death. Iron, coming from the underworld, was considered to be a base metal that needed to be kept isolated from life. Iron was symbolic of harsh, dark, polluted, and hellish strength. Mars is a fiery red planet, and the metal, as well as the god, are associated with fire, war, and conflict.

The mental state induced by *Ferrum metallicum* in persons who have not progressed to a stage of weakness reflects iron's alchemical connection to the planet Mars. When the martial qualities of iron are balanced, they help individuals attain their goals and assert themselves.

When a person has too little of this energy, they are weak and lack of direction. This symptom appears in the homeopathic remedy in the form of spells of weakness, with trembling and a desire to lie down. Walking easily fatigues the individual, and they have loss of strength and feel sleepy during the day. Many of these symptoms are, of course, caused by too little iron in the blood—anemia.

Too much of the warrior quality of Mars causes a stressed and combative attitude toward life. The provings of *Ferrum* reveal its warlike quality. Persons needing iron often have a combative nature. They may be violent, obstinate, and quarrelsome, becoming angry at the least contradiction. Children who need iron often have an iron will and will fight against any attempt on the part of their parents to discipline them. Once these children make up their minds, it is rare that they can be convinced to change them. Because they have not yet learned to suppress their instincts, many of these little one's will get into physical fights with other children and even with adults.

Most adults, on the other hand, channel these tendencies into their work, becoming aggressive, hardworking, and driven. They may be drawn toward the military or become competitive athletes. Others may be managers who rule with an iron hand hidden in a silk glove. In any case, underneath the thin veneer of socialization lies the fiery instinct to do battle. These people may have dreams of battles, fights, and wars, and the individual operates with the underlying premise that life is a battle to be fought and won.

One view of iron, espoused by Anthroposophical medicine, is that iron as a remedy helps to solidify soul and spirit into the physical body, thus shaping the physical body. Without some of the qualities of iron, the body and soul become formless and unable to function in the world.

What is required is a balance that will give the individual enough strength and tension to create the shape of his or her life but not try to hammer it into shape as a blacksmith forms his art.

In either case, whether the fiery energy of Mars is too prominent or underutilized, the homeopathic remedy *Ferrum* can help the individual who is unable to appropriately use this essential aspect of human development. It can bring balance and health by resolving the battle of the opposing forces within the body and mind.

CUPRUM METALLICUM
COPPER

Venus—Love and Beauty

"Love, harmony, and beauty allow life to flow in the right direction."

Cuprum is made from the metal copper, and was first introduced into homeopathy by Samuel Hahnemann. Its well-known homeopathic indications include cramps, spasms, and convulsions. The convulsions often start in the fingers and toes, and many of its ailments are accompanied by blueness, discoloration, and coldness.

Although trace amounts of copper are essential for health, copper in excess can cause depression, arthritis, and hypertension. Smokers and women using the birth control pill are particularly prone to elevated copper levels.

The metal copper gets its name from Cyprus, the island sacred to Venus. Venus, who is associated with love and beauty, would be delighted with the beautiful colors of copper ore, which can be any of a range of vivid colors of blues, greens, reds, and purples. In alchemical literature, copper is also associated with Venus, and the transmutation of copper in inner alchemy has to do with integrating love, sympathy, harmony, and gentleness into consciousness. Since Venus is the planet associated with art, sensory appreciation, and pleasure, the sense of touch is one of the attributes of Venus, as it links physical contact to the emotions with love.

The individual needing copper as a homeopathic remedy not only has physical cramping, but his or her expression of love comes out in a very cramped way. It is as if there is no way for love to be properly expressed or received. The keynote symptom of "worse from touch" indicates how far removed the individual needing this remedy is from the loving physical contact that is an attribute of Venus, the heavenly aspect of the earthly copper.

Most people needing *Cuprum* are very closed and self-critical and have deeply suppressed emotions. In children or adults who have not learned to suppress their emotions, the " cramped" emotions are shown in emotional instability. These people may fly off the handle, be moody, malicious, and be subject to fits of rage. Children needing *Cuprum* can kick and scream, attempt to run away, bite, spit, and be generally nasty.

Those needing *Cuprum* often attempt to channel their cramped emotions by engaging in disciplines such as martial arts or yoga. The martial art is a way of disciplining the aggression, and yoga may temporarily help them feel better because of the amelioration from stretching found in the remedy.

However, because the underlying need to integrate the capacity to give and receive love has not been addressed, these disciplines do not truly help these individuals but rather create a rigid discipline that further removes them from their inner feelings. What should be a flowing and integrating practice often becomes just another way of being cramped. For example, *Cuprum* yoga practitioners often approach this gentle art with a militaristic zeal and discipline that only furthers their tight and cramped body and emotions and often leads to severe injuries.

What is needed is not more discipline or more suppression but some form of help that will open up the constricted emotions and allow the love, pleasure, and harmony associated with the planetary aspect of copper to flow. When the symptoms agree, the combination of the homeopathic remedy *Cuprum* coupled with an understanding of what needs to be healed in the individual may assist them in their journey toward balance and harmony.

MERCURIUS
MERCURY, QUICKSILVER

Mercurius—Communication, the Spirit Imprisoned in Matter
"Communication between the opposites is essential before they can agree on anything."

Mercurius vivus is quicksilver obtained from native mercuric sulfide found in mines. *Mercurius solubilis* is the black oxide of mercury precipitated with *Nitric acid* and ammonia. *Mercurius vivus* and *Mercurius solubilis Hahnemannii* are used in almost the same way and are not differentiated to any degree in most materia medica, although Dutch homeopath Jan Scholten, writes in *Homeopathy and the Elements* that there is a subtle difference between the two. Hahnemann proved both, and some say that he preferred to use *Mercurius vivus*.

Mercury is a poison that affects a wide range of tissues, including mucous membranes, lymph nodes, salivary glands, and especially the nervous system, where it causes neurodegenerative disorders. Because mercury affects the nervous system and accumulates in brain tissue, mercury toxicity is suspected to play a role in the development of Alzheimer's disease. It has also been shown to cause developmental problems and mental retardation in children whose mother's ingested mercury during the fetal and neonatal periods.

As a homeopathic preparation, mercury is considered to be a syphilitic remedy and is well known for ulceration, irritation at night, excessive salivation, night sweats, and sensitivity to both heat and cold.

Because of mercury's ability to dissolve metals and its power to separate gold from impurities, it was of special interest to the alchemists and had much significance in the alchemical process. Mercury symbolized the spirit imprisoned in matter or quintessence, the life-giving vital essence that was thought to exist in all matter. Many alchemical drawings show Mercurius entrapped in a heated, sealed flask symbolizing the transformation that is necessary to release the vital essence. From a psychological point of view, the entrapment and heating of Mercurius represents a withdrawal of projections, a process that definitely turns up the "heat" and forces one to take a closer look at the source of one's difficulties.

However, the quintessence is not the metal quicksilver. Quicksilver was associated with the planet Mercury, the nearest neighbor to the sun and the swiftest planet, ceaselessly spinning in its orbit. This planet was associated with the god Mercurius, also called Hermes, the busy messenger of the gods with wings on his heels, ceaselessly moving from heaven to Earth and from Earth to the underworld. Known also as Thoth in Egypt, he was the god who carried the souls of the dead to the underworld.

Because he constantly carried messages from one realm to another, he represented communication, movement, and adaptation. His constant movements between two realms created a twofold nature. Representing opposing yet complementary principles of light and dark, high and low, male and female, Mercurius contained aspects of evil as well as good.

The homeopathic remedy *Mercurius* also contains this duality. Those needing mercury in its potentized form vacillate back and forth so much that they live in a psychological and physiological state of instability. Dissatisfied about everything around them, they have the delusion that internal turmoil can be alleviated by a change of location. This belief leads to a strong desire to travel, but these people also suffer from homesickness.

Hermes has a good and an evil side, and in the same way, those needing the remedy often have an intense conflict between the desire to create order in a chaotic world and their own violent, destructive impulses. These people often have a desire to maintain peace and a great sensitivity to injustice, as well as a desire to kill and other violent tendencies.

Mercurius is full of contradictory symptoms that are sometimes seen in the same person. It is listed in Kent's repertory under "anarchist or revolutionary," and yet, persons needing this remedy can be very conservative and proper. There is a dichotomy between the mercurial quickness and slowness of mind. An individual requiring this remedy may have a restless, hurried mental state and may not be able to access information. These patients may answer slowly and forget what they wanted to say. It takes them a long time to answer a question, or they speak very quickly and stammer over their words as if their minds cannot quite keep up with their tongue or vice versa.

Everything is too labile. Their minds are easily distracted. While working at one thing another thought comes to mind. These people are constantly distracted by thoughts. Nervous laughter alternates with weeping.

On the physical level, these people often feel great restlessness that is aggravated by the least exertion. Their bodies may tremble, and they may feel sensitivity to both heat and cold. There can be flushes of heat in the face along with icy cold extremities. Heat and chill may alternate.

It is as if the gross metal mercury, with its destructive influence on the nervous system, creates a breakdown in the communication systems of the body and mind. The nervous system gradually loses its ability to make the leap between one synapse and another. The individual is left in a state of duality with no connection, no means of communication between the two extremes.

What is needed is the integration and influence of the heavenly mercury, Hermes with his fleet-footed ability for communication, his ability to move from one sphere to another to heal the rift between the opposites. In other words, what needs to be healed is the lack of communication between the opposites. *Mercurius,* in its homeopathic form, can, as the heavenly mercury symbolizes, open the communication between the opposites and bring the body and mind into greater balance, so the individual no longer need constantly swing between the two.

ARGENTUM METALLICUM
SILVER

The Moon—Wisdom, Soul and the Goddess
"Art must be lead by the muse, not by the nose."

Argentum metallicum was first proved by Hahnemann, who used *Argentum foliatum,* or silver leaf, to prepare the remedy. Silver is known for its effect on cartilage tissue, causing thickening and hardening, for symptoms involving the larynx and vocal cords, and for its characteristic gray discharges.

Repeated exposure to silver dust or fumes can cause the accumulation of large amounts of silver in the body, resulting in kidney damage, lowered fertility, and a blue-gray appearance in the eyes, mucous membranes, and skin.

Silver was associated with the moon and the feminine principle by the alchemists, who considered it to be next to gold in the hierarchy of metals. Silver was thought to be the passive, feminine, and the lunar opposite of the more active, male, and solar metal, gold. In the ultimate merging of opposites, gold and silver as symbols of the great male-female dichotomy must somehow merge to form a greater unity. This is symbolic of the need to develop a perspective that does not deny the presence of good and evil, heaven and Earth, male and female, and other opposites, but rather, one that is able to cope with the reality of the constant existence and interplay of opposing forces as a reality of life.

Silver, is associated with the feminine and the moon, Luna, which has no light of her own, passively reflecting the active male light of the sun with its own white and shining beauty. Luna is associated with the grace of the goddess and the nurturing aspect of Mother Nature. Deeply connected with the unconscious, the moon represents wisdom, timelessness, and potential. The moon is soul. In integrating the heavenly aspect and the earthly aspect of silver, the alchemists were attempting to bring these qualities of the feminine into themselves.

What then does it mean to need silver as a homeopathic remedy? To understand this, it is necessary to look into the parts of the body that are affected by the remedy.

Argentum metallicum primarily affects the cartilage and, in turn, the voice. Cartilage consists of a gelatinous organic matrix in which stiffening collagenous fibers and the matrix-secreting cells are embedded. The resultant mix forms a solid tissue, which is weight bearing and yet quite flexible. Hyaline cartilage is the principal support for the larynx. When healthy, the cartilage of the body is strong and flexible. In the pathology of silver, the cartilage begins to thicken and harden. The individual cannot move about freely and often loses their voice. Other senses, such as hearing and the sense of smell, may become impaired due to a hardening and thickening of the cartilage.

That which is meant to be strong and yet flexible and yielding has become thick and hardened. From a symbolic perspective, the yielding feminine aspect of the individual has not been honored. The soul cannot be expressed.

Argentum metallicum is also known as a remedy for weakness and chronic fatigue. Often the person who needs this remedy has become so weak that it is even difficult for them to tell their symptoms to the homeopath. They look much older than they are. The face is full of wrinkles, and they shy away from company. However, this is in the later stage of their disease.

Before the disease progresses to this stage, these people are often vivacious and sensitive, talkative, and enjoy the company of others. Often they are singers, musicians, speakers, and writers, people who use their mental capacities to express their art or expertise. But they burn out and cannot do it anymore. The burnout happens on the physical level as well as the mental and general level. Along with the symptom of loss of voice in singers there is also writer's cramp. The hardening of the cartilages and the weakness begin to prevent people from expressing themselves.

If we turn back to the alchemists' view of silver and its association to the feminine, we see that these individuals who need *Argentum* have attempted to achieve their goals through the more masculine mental state and have pushed themselves to perform. The more unconscious, passive process of expressing one's art has been confused with the need to push, the need for accomplishment. The more spontaneous expression has been overwhelmed by the need to perform. Thus the well-known symptom of loss of voice in singers is deeply symbolic of the essence of the silver state.

It is not unusual for singers to have trouble with their voices. Ideally, the desire to sing comes from a deep and soulful expression. Singing can express many feelings and can be a transcendental experience. However, the professional singer must sing when they have a performance and must often push themselves beyond the limits of their physical capacities. Because they are always looking for ways to extend the use of the vocal cords, the newest throat remedy or doctor is a great topic of conversation among those who perform with their voice.

When *Argentum metallicum* is needed, the vital force of the individual is creating symptoms of hardness, loss of voice, and eventually deterioration of the cartilage that prevents the person from expressing himself or herself in this forceful and intellectual way. The larynx, which is composed of cartilage, can deteriorate from simple inflammation to paralysis of the vocal cords. If this direction is not changed, the person becomes more and more ossified into the metallic state, unable to even move. There is the typical development of gray discharges. The nervous system may become affected, and there is greater and greater limitation and fatigue.

Homeopathic silver given according to the law of similars can help the individual to integrate the more heavenly, feminine expression within and create a more balanced state of mind and body. It appears that it is necessary for people who need this remedy to sink into the deep, unconscious aspect of their life and allow their muse to guide them.

To allow one's art to flow from the unconscious in a natural way is an ideal that is difficult to attain. The health challenges of those artists needing silver as a homeopathic remedy force them to look for a way of coming closer to this ideal in the expression of their art.

This leaves us with the question as to why some artists can express their work without the need to delve deeply into themselves while others must dive to the depths of their unconscious to retrieve their muse.

AURUM METALLICUM
GOLD

The Sun—the Self, Enlightenment, and Darkness
"The path to enlightenment is like walking the razor's edge."

Aurum metallicum was introduced into the homeopathic materia medica by Hahnemann, who prepared the remedy from pure gold leaf. It is a syphilitic remedy, valued for its effectiveness in treating depression and for heart problems and pains deep in the bones. All symptoms are worse at night, and the pains can be so severe that those needing gold desire death in order to relieve the pain.

Pure gold is nontoxic, but its salts can cause violent gastroenteritis, convulsions, trembling and paralysis. Gold salts produce inflammation and ulceration of connective tissue and mucous membranes and may cause necrosis of the bones. They also act on the central nervous system, causing severe depression.

In Hahnemann's *Materia Medica Pura*, he writes of the early use of gold as a medicine and mentions Geber as an early physician who used gold to rejuvenate the body.[4] Geber, whose true name was Abou Moussah Djafar, was an eighth-century alchemist who wrote much about gold as a medicine, as well as many works on the philosopher's stone and the water of life. Geber thought that a preparation of gold would cure every illness, not only in man but also in all animals and plants. He considered gold to be the only perfect metal, being totally free from "disease."

To Geber, as well as other alchemists, gold was symbolic of the seventh stage of the process of integration of earthly metal with its heavenly, planetary aspect, the sun. It was the final stage of metallic transmutation in preparation for the merging of opposites, or coniunctio, that creates the lapis philosophorum or philosopher's stone.

As with all archetypal symbols, gold has two sides, the shining side that represents the zenith of development and the slide into darkness. Because gold represents eternity, light, power, and riches, its opposite is the total absence of light: darkness, destruction, and suicide.

The level of perfection symbolized by gold, brings with it the perils of such lofty endeavors. The sages who created the *Upanishads* described this danger. They said, "The path to enlightenment is like walking a razor's edge." Jung also warns us about the later stages of development. He writes of the seventh stage of a process as a culmination that brings with it something ominous.

Gold and the sun are both symbolic of the Self, the transpersonal aspect of the individual. According to Jung, the Self is the archetype representing a universal ordering force, but at the same time, it is accessible to human consciousness. The Self is greater than the ego and moves the individual toward wholeness or individuation. The danger in the encounter with the Self is that the individual ego may identify with its transpersonal qualities and become inflated with delusions of grandeur. In order to create balance, there must be a concomitant breaking down of the ego.

The process of breaking down the ego in the seventh stage is often represented in alchemy by the killing of the king. The king with his golden crown must be sacrificed or mortified in order to bring true illumination. He is seen in illustrations being drowned, dismembered, eaten by wolves, or being beheaded. This represents the need for purification from the inflation that is a result of identification with the Self.

From a psychological perspective, this purification is the dark night of the soul or spiritual depression that must be borne in order to integrate the Self, a breaking down of the identification of the ego with the qualities that belong to the god, and can be a very dangerous time because the process entails a kind of death.

The myth of Icarus, who flew too close to the sun, thus melting the wax on his wings and losing his life, is symbolic of inflation and shows its danger. Whenever we fly too high and feel that we can accomplish almost anything, there is compensation from the unconscious to bring us back into balance.

When the compensation for inflation leads to a deep or suicidal depression that is too much for the individual to bear, homeopathic gold, *Aurum metallicum*, may be useful.

As in the symbolism of gold, the individual who needs *Aurum* has a dualistic nature. On one side there is the hardworking, responsible, shining star, the king, and on the other, the darkness into which he can so easily and suddenly slip. We often see the need for *Aurum* in depression, but it is well to recognize the bright side and therefore help the individual to integrate their darker side and avoid the need to fall into a serious and sometimes dangerous downturn.

The symptom "desire to jump from a height" is symbolic of the great fall that may take place when someone constantly drives toward success and identifies with the resultant material rewards, prestige, and accolades. Like those who jumped out of windows during the stock market crash in the 1930s, these people are on very shaky ground. Loss of a business, financial disaster, or humiliation can cause the great fall into a dark depression and a suicidal state.

Aurum contains the dark side of the nature of gold on the physical level as well. *Aurum* is a syphilitic remedy associated with serious disease and destruction of the body. In those who need *Aurum,* there may be a tendency to heart and vascular problems, severe headaches, and destruction of the bones. The pains, which are mostly worse at night, may be so severe as to drive the person to suicide or to take powerful narcotic drugs.

Many people needing *Aurum,* like King Midas who wished for everything around him to turn into gold, are attached to the material world. Others simply identify with the positive, hardworking, or religious aspect of their nature, choosing to ignore the darker side until a serious depression drops them into a pit of despair. Others tempt fate from time to time, discharging the underlying darkness by risking their lives. These people drive in a fast and dangerous way, especially when they are angry, or they may participate in dangerous sports such as mountain climbing, where they take unnecessary risks.

The sun, as a heavenly body, is the symbol of authority, the father, and the paternal influence on the psyche, in the form of training, education, discipline, and morality. It stands for social constraint and censorship that can crush the individual with rules and prejudices, but it also is the source of a higher image of the self that can be an inspiration to move forward in life.

We see this influence in children who need *Aurum.* They are considered to be very special and may be gifted. Serious about their studies, they want to be the best in their class and push themselves very hard. There are far too many golden children, because these qualities are seen as very positive and desirable. Instead of being guided into a more balanced way of life, they are encouraged to continue their striving by schools, teachers, and parents who bask in the light of their success. They excel at everything they do and are far too serious and successful. One slip, one failed exam, is all that it takes, and down they go. It makes one wonder if *Aurum* was needed by the Japanese children, who, failing to get into the best kindergarten, committed suicide.

The overly responsible and moral nature of the gold personality can turn into irresponsibility and immorality. This change may occur after a disappointed love affair or other disappointments because of which the person becomes hardened, shuts out all possibilities for love, and develops deep hatred and animosity. Violent outbursts of anger, acts of violence, and other antisocial behavior can accompany this state. People with this personality may also turn toward alcoholism and drug addiction, especially to the use of LSD and other hallucinogenic drugs. Although *Aurum* is more commonly known for its value in treating the internalized violence of suicide, the darkness and violence in those who are farther along in the pathology treated by *Aurum* can also be projected outward onto the environment.

In both children and adults, *Aurum* can help to avoid the need to permanently fall into the darkness. This remedy acts deeply and can help in some of the most serious and painful physical and mental diseases. Indeed, as described by the alchemist Geber, it is a wonderful substance capable of rejuvenating the body. Moreover, as homeopaths, we may add, it is a great healer of the mind and soul, as well as the body.

CHAPTER FIFTEEN

The Internal Saboteur

Some people do not respond to a seemingly well-indicated homeopathic remedy. This lack of response has been an object of discussion in homeopathic circles ever since Hahnemann first contemplated this problem and came up with the role of miasms in chronic disease.

The following chapter covers a group of remedies that are of value for a particular category of resistance to healing. These remedies are indicated for persons who have a history of severe trauma due to abuse or lack of adequate nurturance in their childhood. The trauma may also originate later in life and be actual or perceived. Whatever the cause, the only way that these individuals were able to survive unbearable pain was by disassociation.

In these situations, part of the psyche has been split off, and an entity within the inner state is created in order to protect the essence or self of the traumatized individual. I call this part the internal saboteur, because it resists any outside attempt to change the status quo of the individual whom it protects. It has developed a life of its own and is a bodyguard that cannot differentiate between an assassin and a friend.

Whenever the individual makes any attempt to heal this entity creates a powerful resistance. Neither well-meaning therapist nor physician is allowed to interfere in the mechanisms that were established long ago and served to protect the person from the initial trauma. Even though these individuals very much want to get well, it is as if they are possessed by a demon that overrides their conscious desires.

Many psychotherapists have recognized this phenomenon in patients who were particularly resistant to treatment. Freud named it the diamonic resistance or severe superego, and Jung saw it as possession by a complex. Donald Kalsched, who explores this subject in depth in his book *The Inner World of Trauma*, refers to it as the self-care system:

> *The self-care system performs the self-regulatory and inner/outer me-*
> *diational functions that, under normal conditions, are performed by the*
> *person's functioning ego. Here is where a problem arises. Once the trauma*
> *defense is organized, all relations with the outer world are "screened" by*
> *the self-care system. What was intended to be a defense against further*
> *trauma becomes a major resistance to all unguarded spontaneous expres-*
> *sions of self in the world.*[1]

Whatever its name, this state is characterized by an extreme and unconscious resistance to therapy of any kind and can lead to great difficulty in
finding the correct remedy. The presence of the internal saboteur may be
recognized by the lack of response or extreme aggravation of symptoms
when a well-indicated remedy is administered. Mostly invisible, the internal
saboteur appears symbolically in violent dreams of dismemberment, mutilation, and other forms of self-destruction. It can appear as a frightening
and dominating figure and even sometimes convert itself into a more benevolent protective form. These dreams often appear after a remedy has had
a deep and healing effect and the individual begins to move away from
ingrained patterns of behavior.

Whether in the frightening or more benevolent form, dreams of the
internal saboteur have an ominous quality about them, as they are an attempt to prevent any interference with the defense system.

The internal saboteur can also be felt by the homeopath as a deep resistance to treatment. One finds oneself walking on eggshells, being careful
not to offend by the slightest comment. Even taking the greatest care, the
homeopath may become embroiled in a very difficult situation. When this
happens, homeopaths should look into their own psychic states and attempt to discriminate between their internal dynamics and those of the
client. Given this, when the homeopath still has a strong feeling of aversion
or frustration, it may be a clue to the presence of the internal saboteur.

Recognition of the cause is the first step in finding the most effective
remedy. It is important to understand that an intercurrent remedy (a remedy that is given when the indicated remedy stops working) may be needed—
one for the whole person and one for the saboteur. However, the same
remedy may cover the entire case.

When no characteristic symptoms are obvious, the type of disease may
give a clue to the presence of the internal saboteur. Autoimmune disorders,
which are characterized by a misdirected immune response in which the
body's defenses become self-destructive, are the bodily mirror of this

phenomenon. It is as if the autoimmune disease is a somatization of the psychic process—with what should be an immune response taking over and creating disease.

In a normally functioning immune system, recognition of self is accomplished through the major histocompatibility complex (MHC). Although the entire process is not understood, in the case of autoimmunity, the immune system is unable to recognize what is self (normal tissue and fluid) and what is nonself (invading organisms and toxins). The same confusion of what is self and what is nonself is present in many people with a history of severe trauma.

Other types of diseases in which this "attacking force/self-care system" within the psyche may come into play are immune disorders such as immune system hypersensitivity (allergic disorders, antibody-dependent cytotoxicity) and diseases such as candidiasis, in which cells mutate or overtake the organism.

Unconscious repetition of traumatic events throughout the person's life, as well as internal conflicts, may also be a key to the remedy. As Kalsched describes, possession by this split-off part of the psyche tends to replicate the initial trauma in the inner and outer world of the individual:

> *The first of these findings ... [in literature exploring the inner world of trauma] is that the traumatized psyche is self-traumatizing. Trauma doesn't end with the cessation of outer violation, but continues unabated in the inner world of the trauma victim, whose dreams are often haunted by persecutory inner figures. The second finding is the seemingly perverse fact that the victim of psychological trauma continually finds himself or herself in life situations where he or she is re-traumatized. As much as he or she wants to change, as hard as he or she tries to improve life or relationships, something more powerful than the ego continually undermines progress and destroys hope. It is as though the persecutory inner world somehow finds its outer mirror in repeated self-defeating "re-enactments" —almost as if the individual were possessed by some diabolical power or pursued by a malignant fate.[2]*

Carefully analysis of the repetitive pattern may lead to an understanding of what remedy is indicated. This type of analysis can be useful if there are few or no characteristic symptoms in other areas of the case or if the characteristic symptoms lead to a remedy which has been given and failed to get results. For example: A woman comes to homeopathic treatment for arthritis and has had much previous medical care. Each medicine she receives makes her worse, and she is treated very badly by all of the practitioners she has seen. She feels that they have abused her. Her anamnesis shows a great amount of abuse from an early age and a history of cruel relationships. She is given *Calcarea carbonica* because her physical, general, and even most of her mental symptoms point to this remedy. Instead of getting better on the remedy, she is terribly aggravated by it and feels that the homeopath, like all of her other practitioners, is mistreating her.

If the case is analyzed in light of a repetitive pattern trauma, the relevant symptoms may be seen in the continuation of the early childhood abuse. As a child, her parents, on whom she was dependent, abused her. She married and was abused by her husband, on whom she was dependent, and continued this pattern in later relationships with men. After the onset of arthritis, she turned to health-care practitioners, relying on their expertise for help, and when her condition was aggravated by their medicine, she felt personally abused by them.

Based on the repetitive pattern, the indicated remedy may be *Lyssin*, because of the repetitive pattern of "those on whom I depend abuse me."

The following materia medica is based on remedies that may be considered in cases in which there is a history of severe childhood trauma and well-indicated remedies fail to work. It begins with the remedy *Lyssin*, which I consider to be one of the most important remedies in this arena. Many of these remedies are helpful as intercurrent remedies, to be given when the indicated remedy works for a time and suddenly becomes ineffective.

LYSSIN
THE INTERNAL SABOTEUR

Lyssin is a nosode, or a homeopathic remedy made from a disease product, prepared by the American homeopath Constanine Hering from the saliva of a rabid dog. Also called *Hydrophobinum, Lyssin* was proved by Hering in 1833. He subsequently made a complete pathogenesis of hydrophobia, or rabies, in sixty pages of his *Guiding Symptoms*. Hering thought the saliva contained venom, although we now know a virus causes rabies.

The symbolism of the dog appears in many cultures as the psychopomp, the spirit who guides souls to the underworld. Dogs also appear as the intermediary between the two worlds; the world of the living and the world of the dead. Many cultures bury dogs along with dead people so that the dogs may guide the soul to the place of the dead.

Because *Lyssin* is made from the saliva of a rabid dog, it is symbolically related to dangerous and fierce dogs, Cerberus being one of the most famous. Cerberus is the mythical monstrous dog with three heads and a dragon's tail that guards the gates of hell, barring it to the living and preventing the dead from escaping. Hercules's final and most dangerous task was to descend into the underworld and conquer this beast. Encountering monsters and ghosts along the journey, he made his way to Hades, where he found Pluto, the god of the underworld. Pluto agreed that Hercules could capture Cerberus and bring him to the surface if he could overpower the beast with his own brute strength.

Hercules agreed and, finding Cerberus at the gates of one of the five rivers of the underworld, Hercules wrestled Cerberus into submission, even though the dragon in the tail of the flesh-eating dog bit him. Ignoring the pain, Hercules brought Cerberus to the surface, where saliva fell from the mouth of the monster onto the earth and gave birth to the plant aconite. Later, Hercules, having fulfilled his last task, returned Cerberus to Hades, where he continues to guard the gateway of the underworld.

To conquer Cerberus represents descending into a personal hell and facing whatever demons dwell there. In the case of an individual who needs *Lyssin*, there is often a confrontation with an indwelling spirit that must be integrated into the conscious state. As the hound of hell, Cerberus symbolizes the terrors of death and the hell within each individual. A hell that is mirrored in the physical and emotional state of *Lyssin* has been caused by the experience of violence and abuse.

Those who require *Lyssin* have experienced a hell that is guarded by Cerberus, and with the help of the remedy, they must once more descend into the depths of their unconscious and bring their trauma back to the surface of the conscious mind. This is not an easy task, but given enough spiritual strength and guidance, it can be done. Many times, the psyche has been split into pieces and the guard at the door bars entrance to all but the most persevering. Cerberus is there for a reason, and he will put up a fight. The following symptoms in this section are from Hering's *Guiding Symptoms*.[3]

> *Declares amid violent sobs that she is suffering the torments of hell.*

Contemporary homeopaths have begun to use this remedy in cases where there is a severe trauma from childhood abuse. *Lyssin* is an important intercurrent remedy when well-indicated remedies stop working and there are elements of extreme violence in the individual or in the family history. In persons requiring *Lyssin*, the violence experienced in the past is often turned inward and is expressed as self-mutilation.

> *Insane ideas enter his head; for instance, to throw a glass of water, which he is carrying in his hand, into someone's face, or to stab his flesh with the knife he is holding, and the like.*

> *Ordered her husband to go away, as she wanted to bite him, and joining act to threat, she bit herself in arm.*

These symptoms of self-mutilation are also indications of conflicting energies existing within the psyche. These have been called various names. Freud named these conflicting energies the diamonic resistance or severe superego, and Jung saw it as possession by a complex. In shamanism, this resistant part of the spirit was diagnosed as possession by a spirit or soul loss. Along with the more obvious symptoms of self-mutilation, it may manifest in the body as types of disorders that are particularly resistant to all types of treatment. This resistance may be within the nature of the psychic disturbance, for it is has been put into place very early in life to protect the essence or self of the individual during early childhood trauma. What was once a defense that was necessary for survival of the child now stands, as Cerberus guards the gate, in the way of healing, and persons with this "self-care system" will often respond in a negative way to even the gentlest of treatments.[4]

This self-care system or internal saboteur can also cause a split in the personality. The individual will choose one way, but the internal saboteur has taken on a life of its own and often opposes the conscious will. This tendency was experienced in Hering's proving of *Lyssin*.

> *It seems to her as if two entirely different trains of thought influenced her at the same time.*

In the case of autoimmune disease there are often a strong forces within the psyche that attack and prevent healing from taking place. It is as if the autoimmune disease is a somatization of this process, with what should be an immune response taking over and creating disease. This attacking force within the psyche may come into play in immune disorders such as immune system hypersensitivity. In many of these cases, we may need to give a remedy such as *Lyssin* for the fundamental characteristic of the disease— the organism attacking itself.

In myth and symbolism, powers of divination, second sight, and healing are attributed to the dog, and we see these symptoms in *Lyssin*. It is found under the heading "clairvoyance" in Kent's *Repertory of the Homeopathic Materia Medica,* and Knerr's extraction of Hering's work includes the symptom *"Sympathetic, felt same pain his brother complained of."* Not only do these people experience the suffering of their own hell, they experience the sufferings of others as well. This proving symptom gives us a clue that these people may experience trauma through the sufferings of others. Given this, one could expect that the *Lyssin* state could come about in sensitive or even clairvoyant people who are exposed to violence and trauma experienced by others.

The feeling of abuse and trauma that they carry within themselves is projected outward, continuing the cycle of abuse in their lives.

> *Imagine that they are being abused, and energetically defend themselves against attacks and insults, which in reality are products of their own fancy.*

From the very beginning, the alchemists worked with the symbol of the dog, including the mating of dogs, which symbolically indicated the merging of two substances. For our purpose, one of the most interesting alchemical references is to the mad dog and to hydrophobia:

> *This Chamaeleon is the infant hermaphrodite, who is infected from his very cradle by the bite of the Corascene dog, whereby he is maddened and rages with perpetual hydrophobia; nay, though of all natural things water is the closest to him, yet he is terrified of it and flees from it.*[5]

Jung comments on this paragraph. "It is clear," he says, "that this refers to a psychic disturbance which at one stage also infected the 'infant hermaphrodite.'. . . Just how the mad dog with its terror got into the water at all is not clear, unless it was in the water from the very beginning."

As homeopaths, we recognize the phenomenon of the rabies miasm, which is passed down from generation to generation; that's how it got into the water. In reading this passage, one has to wonder if the alchemist who wrote it was directly intuiting the *Lyssin* miasm. He certainly is accurate in its rage and in the well-known symptom of *Lyssin,* fear of water.

ALUMINA
WHO AM I?

Alumina is aluminum hydroxide or clay and is the main ingredient of many gemstones, including ruby, emerald sapphire, topaz, and amethyst.

Hahnemann introduced it into the homeopathic materia medica. The remedy is known to be a difficult one to prescribe, because the people requiring it have difficultly expressing themselves. They are very confused as to who they really are (confusion as to identity) and, therefore, cannot clearly describe themselves in a way that differentiates themselves from others. This remedy is most often given based on slowness of mind and body. People requiring this remedy must think a long time before answering a question and are often confused. The body processes are slow, particularly peristalsis, leading to the well-known keynote symptom of obstinate constipation with soft stool. This slowness and confusion, combined with pervasive dryness, are often the only symptoms on which homeopaths can base their prescription.

Alumina is a very ordinary, innocuous substance, clay, which has the ability to mold itself into many shapes and forms. In its more exalted state it becomes a gemstone. Because of its ability to be molded into any shape, *Alumina* contains the capacity for infinite possibilities. Like clay, the *Alumina* personality, while suffering from a lack of identity, has the possibility of going beyond where those with a more rigid structure can go. Those who need this remedy can, if treated in the earlier states of the disease, become gemstones. They have the capacity to develop that gem of priceless value, the philosopher's stone. The philosopher's stone is the ultimate goal of the alchemist's opus and, from a psychological point of view, represents individuation. The stone is found, the alchemists say, on garbage heaps and in excrement. It is at once rare and the most common of material.

Like the philosopher's stone that lays hidden in common and base material, persons needing *Alumina* often have a deep inner life, which, when uncovered in the healing process, reveals great treasure. In order to reveal these gifts, however, they must cut through and eliminate aspects of their psychic landscape. These are aspects of their psyche where they have identified with others to the extent that the individual psyche is dominated by outside influences. In the case of deep trauma, these psychic personages can be the perpetrators of abuse or, if the family of origin is seriously dysfunctional, it could be identification with family members. Because the people who need *Alumina* are so malleable, they seem to be able to absorb the psychic state of others to the degree that they lose themselves completely.

In the *Alumina* state, the "false self" or internal saboteur is not formed into a single entity but continually shifts. In other remedy states, the traumatized individual completely identifies with the false self and therefore has a sense of identity, albeit one that is not the true self. These false inner beings with which the *Alumina* patient identifies must be eliminated for the true nature to shine through. During this process there may be dreams of shooting or stabbing people and other expressions of violence that are uncharacteristic of the conscious state. This is the meaning of this symptom found in the old provings: "Seeing blood on a knife she has horrid ideas of killing herself, though she abhors the idea." [6] Dreams such as these may indicate the need for the remedy or may appear as a positive response after the remedy is given. In any case, it is a clear example of a dream functioning as the psyche's attempt to heal the individual.

ABSINTHIUM
THE GREEN FAIRY

Absinthium is made from *Artemesia absinthium*, or wormwood. It should not be confused with *Artemesia vulgaris*, which is also called wormwood. Wormwood is one of the major ingredients of the infamous liqueur absinthe, which was a favorite of many writers and artists, including Oscar Wilde, Ernest Hemingway, and Vincent van Gogh. Absinthe reportedly acted as an aphrodisiac, and intoxication with absinthe was said to inspire the creative muse. Because of these attributes and its green color, it became known as the "green fairy." Absinthe soon became illegal because of its toxic effects, which included delusions and peculiar epileptic-like symptoms. Since it was a favorite drink of van Gogh's, one wonders if many of his problems were caused by absinthe or if he actually needed it in its potentized form. He painted many of his works in ochre and pale greens, which are the colors of absinthe, and many of his self-portraits are of him seated at a bar with glasses of the aperitif.

Absinthium was proved by Dr. H. P. Gatchell, but many of the known symptoms come from known poisonings with the liqueur. According to Frans Vermeulen,[7] a modern proving was done in 1988 by Gruppe Dynamis with nine provers.

The characteristic physical symptoms showing a need for *Absinthium* are listed in John Henry Clarke's *A Dictionary of Practical Materia Medica* as the following:

> *Convulsions preceded by trembling, the patient makes grimaces, bites tongue, foams. Vertigo on rising, with a tendency to fall backward and epileptoid attacks of hysterical character with tremors and opisthotonos. Tremors, tremor of tongue, of the heart. The patient is obliged to walk around.*

The mental symptoms indicating the need for the remedy have some of the qualities so desired by the drinker of absinthe. The person feels as if he or she is going into a beautiful dream and is very tranquil, feeling as if the brain were rounded and symmetrical. However, the largest number of symptoms indicate a state of cold, unfeeling brutality:

> *Insane, idiotic, brutal. Idiotic manner doesn't care whether she dies or not. Stupor alternating with dangerous violence.*[8]

These symptoms may be experienced on a conscious level, or, in the case of a person who has been exposed to much trauma, can emerge from the unconscious in the form of strange dreams and symptoms that are characteristic of the internal saboteur.

Many forms of hallucinations and visions can also show up in dreams. People requiring *Absinthium* are full of frightful visions and terrifying hallucinations. The patient may have hallucinations of people pursuing him or her; or the patient may see all kinds of animals, cats and rats of all colors, grotesque animals, or demons.

As the internal defense mechanism can also threaten the life of the individual rather than allow interference or change in the defenses that have been put in place, it is not uncommon for people requiring *Absinthium* to feel a sensation that death is imminent or that they are is about to be killed. In *Absinthium* patients, we often find fear of assassination.

ACONITUM NAPELLUS
SHAKEN BY FEAR

Aconitum napellus, commonly known as aconite, monkshood, or wolfbane, was first introduced into the homeopathic materia medica by Hahnemann. It is prepared from the root and whole plant when it is beginning to flower. This well-known remedy is commonly used for acute fright and panic, first stages of colds and flu, and high fevers that come on suddenly. Sudden onset and intensity of symptoms are keynotes of the remedy, as is the aggravation of symptoms from cold wind.

More recently, George Vithoulkas has introduced its use in more chronic conditions characterized by deep fear and anxiety. *Aconitum napellus* is a remedy to think of whenever there are symptoms that have never been well since a great fright, so it is an important remedy in situations of childhood trauma.

Aconite has a mythological connection to Cerberus, the dog who guards the gates of hell. It is said that when Hercules conquered the many-headed

Cerberus by overcoming him through brute strength, the saliva from Cerberus's mouth fell to the ground and from that sprang aconite. Through this myth we see the relationship between *Lyssin*, made from the saliva of a mad dog, and *Aconitum.*

In practice, it is not unusual for someone who has been riddled with fear caused by trauma to need one of these remedies followed by the other. The two remedies complement one another well. *Aconitum*, with its associated symptoms of self-torture and antagonism to oneself, indicates the presence of the internal saboteur. This remedy is especially helpful when symptoms of early fright and terror are uncovered in the healing process and now dominate the dreams and even the waking life of the individual.

AGARICUS MUSCARIUS
THE FEARFUL WARRIOR

Agaricus muscarius or *Amanita muscarius* is a mushroom, with a showy scarlet red or orange cap and white spots, found growing over most of North America, Asia, and Europe. It was proved by Hahnemann, the full proving appearing in his *Chronic Diseases.* This mushroom is well known for its use in frostbite, facial twitching, sciatica, and anxiety about health, and the provings indicate a much more intense mental state. Farokh Masters, contemporary homeopath and author of *Fascinating Fungi*, describes *Agaricus* as an important remedy in the treatment of alcoholism.

This mushroom is an intoxicant and in some cases a hallucinogen. It was taken by Siberian shamans to attain a state of ecstasy. Mircea Eliade mentions the use of *Agaricus* among Indo-European shamans in his authoritative text *Shamanism: Archaic Techniques of Ecstasy.* The alkaloids in the mushroom create an ecstatic state, with much hilarity and increased strength.

Individuals needing *Agaricus* have an overwhelming fear of death and may wake up at night terrified by this fear. Their connection with death is accompanied by metaphysical speculation about what death would be like and what happens after death. Because of this and their extreme anxiety about health, these people are often drawn to the healing professions, especially those healing arts which combine science and metaphysics.

These people are often clairvoyant, and their fascination with death can be accompanied by premonitions. They take solace in helping others to have a peaceful demise.

People who need *Agaricus* often display symptoms of mutilation and violence, indicating the presence of the internal saboteur. The patient may have a desire to mutilate his or her body and show a fearless, threatening, destructive frenzy that may turn inward or be expressed in violent acts. During this time the individual may be extremely destructive and exhibit superhuman strength. Especially when under the influence of alcohol or cocaine, the individual is capable of tearing up cars, breaking down doors, and smashing through plate glass.

A delusion that he or she is under superhuman control, is one possible symptom, usually a projection of the internal state of the individual. This symptom is a conflict caused by having one part of the psyche dominating the will. This may become so unbearable that it cannot be contained and must be projected outward onto the environment. The individual then believes that demons or persons are attempting to control his or her life.

Symptoms exhibited by the inner conflict may be acted out and experienced on a bodily level or conscious mental state, but more frequently they are seen through dreams and symbolic physical symptoms. Examples of the physical symptoms that relate to the inner feeling of torture are severe and debilitating pains in the back emanating from the spine. These are often caused by herniation of the spinal discs. *Agaricus* is a leading remedy for this problem. If violent dreams of mutilation accompany these physical symptoms and well-indicated remedies fail to help, this mushroom may be the answer.

FOLLICULINUM
PATRIARCHAL DOMINATION OF THE FEMININE

Folliculinum is a potentized form of natural estrogen, first prepared in the 1950s by the Scottish homeopath Donald Foubister. Foubister suggests that if well-indicated remedies fail to act for a patient undergoing extreme pressure, *Folliculinum* may be indicated, at least until the pressures are past. Although there is no Hahnemannian proving of *Folliculinum* at this time, Othon A. Julian, author of *Materia Medica of New Homeopathic Remedies*, reports extensive clinical indications for this remedy.

Physical symptoms include premenstrual migraines, prolonged and painful menses, mettrorhagia, and swelling of the breasts. The woman generally feels worse before her menses, during ovulation, and when she becomes overheated. The mental symptoms include moods alternating between excitability and depression that are worse before menses, sexual hyperexcitability, and fixed ideas pertaining to sex. Extreme mental instability with anguish was also part of the clinical picture.

Bruno Marinez, M.D., conducted a survey, published in the *British Homoeopathic Journal*, of thirty-two patients treated with *Folliculinum* for premenstrual syndrome that showed an 88 percent response to overall improvement and a 100 percent improvement in metrorrhagia.[9] In addition, in an impressive paper in the same journal, Dorothy J. Cooper reports the results of her work with *Folliculinum* over twenty years involving nearly three hundred patients and over seven hundred prescriptions.[10]

Ms. Cooper confirms Foubister's suggestion that persons undergoing extreme pressure may require *Folliculinum*. She has seen three categories of pressure that may indicate the need for this remedy. The first is when a dominant parent, friend, or spouse pressures an individual. Also in this category is pressure exerted by intolerant religious groups. The second category is when the individual has worked himself or herself to the point of exhaustion over a period of time and even well-indicated remedies fail to work. The third is the pressure of chronic ill health after recurrent or severe infection. These are individuals who have a diagnosis of "post-viral syndrome" or "chronic fatigue syndrome."

Although 15 percent of Cooper's patients were men, *Folliculinum* is primarily a remedy for women. It is important in menopause, not only because of its excellent result in treating hot flashes and metrorrhagia but also because its indication of "domination from others" helps to free the woman from the insidious and underlying domination caused by living in a patriarchal society.

In modern-day Western society, many women experience the emergence of the internal saboteur around menopause. They have internalized society's demand for a youthful appearance and attitude and often experience the onset of menopause as a loss of identity. This attitude amounts to a miasm that has been imprinted on women, and on the female side of men. *Folliculinum* can help to remove this miasm and free the feminine nature from the domination of the patriarchal saboteur.

LILIUM TIGRINUM
SUPPRESSION OF EROS

Lilium tigrinum was introduced into homeopathy by Dr. W. E. Payne, who conducted a proving of it under the supervision of Carroll Dunham. Most of the provers were women doctors. Some of the provings were made with remedies made from the pollen of the tiger lily, while others were done with remedies made from the tincture of fresh stalks, leaves, and flowers of the plant. One of the woman provers was under Dunham's direct supervision at the time of the proving and he gives his account of the case in his *Science of Therapeutics:*

> Lilium tigrinum *is primarily a woman's remedy, having a strong effect on the female sexual organs. On the physical level there are bearing down sensations in the uterus, pains in the ovarian region, and thin acrid leucorrhoea that leaves a brown stain. Sexual desire is very strong, and on the emotional level, there is much conflict between the individual's passionate nature and her religious beliefs.*

The symbol of the lily itself also contains this dichotomy. The lily symbolizes heavenly purity, innocence, and virginity, but also represents love and passion. In the biblical tradition, the lily represented the mystical surrender to the will of god, but Greek mythology relates the lily to unlawful passion. Because of the phallic pistils emerging from the open trumpet shape of the petals, lilies are considered symbols of procreation.

The tiger lily, which combines the purity of the lily with its orange and black tigerlike coloring, inspires the imagination toward eroticism. A research on tiger lily on the Internet reveals that many women involved in the erotic arts have taken on the name of this flower.

As a homeopathic remedy, *Lilium tigrinum* exhibits the split in the personality so often found when there is early childhood trauma. Here the split is between the powerful forces of sexuality and spirituality, which creates great anxiety and restlessness. There is a great sense of hurriedness, a desire to escape from the sexual feelings, which cause so much conflict. In his *Encyclopedia of Pure Materia Medica*, Allen writes the following:

> *Constant hurried feeling as of imperative duties and utter inability to perform them; during the sexual excitement.*

> *The sexual desire, dormant hitherto, was so strongly aroused that the prover said, "I am afraid of myself, I seem possessed of a demon."*[11]

The demon that she is tormented by is the conflict between internalized religious ideas and her sexual passions. It implies the presence of a destructive religious influence within the psyche that denies the spiritual validity of her sexuality. Many religions have negativity toward sexuality and impose guilt upon their followers, but the person requiring *Lilium* has absorbed guilt about sexuality into his or her being. These individuals have a great vulnerability to being wounded in this way, either because of a basic sensitivity or because of early childhood sexual trauma. Sometimes, it is enough for a sensitive child to simply hear of sexual abuse to be traumatized; for others there must be more obvious abuse in order to create the imprint. Whatever the cause, the guilt around sexuality and sexual feelings are in conflict with the individual's deeply felt religious tendencies to the point that the person feels tormented. Constantine Hering, in his *Guiding Symptoms*, writes that woman with these symptoms is "tormented about her salvation."

This restlessness and torment is accompanied by violent anger and the desire to swear and curse. The individual is depressed and weeps, grieving over what has happened or searching for something to grieve over. When confronted with their behavior, these individuals can become violent and throw things or hit people. A prover reported:

> *While attending a lecture (speech), desire to hit the lecturer, and in the evening desirous of swearing and damning the fire and things generally, and to think and speak obscene things; disposed to strike and hit persons; as these feelings came, the uterine pains passed away.*[12]

This behavior, which the individual cannot control, aggravates the patient's mood, making the patient feel even more separated from himself or herself. It is as if there are two people and the violent one is tormenting the patient.

In its potentized form, the beautiful tiger lily may help a person in this state to live a healthier and happier life. In order to assist in this healing, it is important for the homeopath to understand how deep the wound is that causes this type of split in the psyche. It may even be necessary to give other remedies along the way in order to facilitate the healing process.

Other Remedies for the Internal Saboteur

Many remedies besides the ones previously mentioned might be useful in the treating people who have been severely traumatized. The purpose of this list is to point to certain remedies that may be indicated in these cases and jog the mind to think about other possibilities.

The following remedies have symptoms indicative of their use in cases where there is a split in the personality or the presence of a conflicting or destructive energy within the psyche (internal saboteur). They may be useful when well-indicated remedies fail to produce results or in autoimmune diseases. Remedies that indicate that they are a polychrest belonging to a certain group, for instance, *Lachesis* (snake polychrest) means that the remedy represents a well-known remedy within a particular family of remedies. In these cases, it is worth looking into the other remedies in that group that are less well known. For instance, *Lachesis* is a well-known snake remedy and has many indications for this differential. Other lesser-known snake remedies may also have these symptoms.

Absinthium: Hallucination of vision and of hearing, that he is pursued by imaginary enemies. Sees terrifying animals, cats and rats of all colors. Hyperactivity, cannot stop in one place because of horrible visions that come to her. Brutal. Dangerous violence. Fear of assassination.

Aconite: Antagonism with herself—self-torture. Alternate attacks of opposite moral symptoms.

Agaricus: Delusion he is under superhuman control. Inclination to mutilate his body. He becomes so furious that he can hardly be restrained from ripping up his bowels, as he fancies the mushroom had ordered him to do. Fearless, threatening, destructive frenzy, also such as turns against itself and injures itself, combined with great exertion of strength.

Alcoholus: Various hallucinations of sight, hearing, smell, and sensation. Thinks he is pursued by robbers, murderers, police, etc. Melancholy with inclination to commit suicide.

Alumina: Delusion head belongs to another, head separated from body. Sees anything as if another person had seen it or as if he could transfer himself into another and only then could see. She cannot see blood or a knife without horrible thoughts pressing upon her, as if she should commit suicide; though she has the greatest horror of it.

Ambra Grisea: Distorted fancies, satanic faces take possession of the mind and he cannot get rid of them.

Anacardium: Delusion devil in one ear angel in other; possessed; as if under superhuman control. Hears voices that he must follow. Possessed of two wills. Delusion head separated from body and thoughts are separated. Fixed ideas—that strange forms accompany him, one to his right, and one to his left. Antagonism with himself. Delusion he is dead, is surrounded by enemies.

Androctonus: It seems as though he was a different person, very similar to the way he had been in adolescence but in a more powerful manner.

These emotions were so intense he wanted to rip his chest apart and let them out. He lost all control over his emotions, which seemed to come from a deep, distant part of himself, a darker side.

Arsenicum: Inclination to mutilate his body. Self-torture. Torments himself. Continued anxiety, a mental anguish, as if he had not done his duty, without, however, knowing wherein. Became very nervous, agitated, and delirious, suspecting people were about the house plotting against his life, jumps out of bed and suddenly reaches after imaginary objects.

Antimonium tartaricum: Delusion that his head is separated from his body. Antagonism with himself. Contradiction between mind and will.

Aurum metallicum: Antagonism with herself, contemptuous of self. He thinks that he everywhere finds an impediment, caused now by an opposing fate, then again by himself, which later mortifies him and renders him detected.

Belladonna: Delusion possessed. Inclination to mutilate his body. Self-torture. Torments himself. She tries to strangle herself and begs the bystanders to kill her because she believes that she will certainly die. Delusions and visions of horrible, frightening animals.

Candida albicans: Delusion surrounded by enemies.

Cannabis indicus: Delusion he is bewitched; possessed of the devil. Astonished to find themselves not masters of their own will. Delusion, body is divided; head belongs to another; head separated from body. Delusion, mind and body are separated; soul is separated from the body. Antagonism with herself.

Cantharis: Delusion, possessed; as if seized. Visions . . . something took hold of her hand, and bent it several times up and down, then it seemed as if someone took her by the throat with ice-cold hands.

Camphora: Delusion he is dead. As I lay stretched on my couch, as the evil demon, and suffered all the anguish of a condemned and God-forsaken soul . . . I was forever deprived of Divine protection and of every consolation and every hope. The child creeps into a corner, howls and cries; everything that is said to him is taken as if one was ordering him, and he was considered naught and should be punished.

Crotalus horridus: Delusion body is only half alive. Aversion to himself. Imagines himself surrounded by enemies or hideous animals.

Folliculinum: Delusion she is under a powerful influence. Ailments from domination. She feels controlled by another; has no identity.

Germanium: Delusion every movement and thought is controlled; is under a powerful influence. Delusion hand is separated from her body. I picture myself lying on floor in fetal position and being shot in the head like a horse or a dog.

Hyoscyamus: Delusion possessed by the devil; is under a powerful influence; possessed; as if seized. Delusion mind and body are separated. Inclination to mutilate his body.

Kali bromatum: Thinks he is pursued, will be poisoned, and is selected for divine vengeance.

Lac caninum (milk polychrest): Delusion she has someone else's nose. Antagonism with herself. Aversion to herself. Contemptuous of self. Is impressed with the idea that all she says is a lie; it seems to be very difficult to speak the truth, but continually distrusts things. Woke at daylight feeling that she is a loathsome, horrible mass of disease, could not bear to look at any portion of her body. Sensation or delusion as if surrounded by myriads of snakes.

Lachesis (snake polychrest): Delusion, charmed, cannot break the spell, is under a powerful influence, as if under superhuman control. Hears voices he must follow, possessed of two wills. Antagonism with herself. Delusion he is dead. Thinks she is somebody else, in the hands of a stronger power.

Lilium tigrinum: The sexual desire was so strong that the prover said, "I am afraid of myself, I seem possessed of a demon." Delusion body is divided. Self-torture. Torments himself. Perceptive and reflexive faculties seem benumbed, whereas at first she was overactive and seemed to be two individuals.

Lycopodium: Aversion to herself. Desire to look only on the bright (light) side of life. Fear of looking into the dark side of life.

Lyssin: Antagonism with herself. Impulse to stab himself with a knife. Two distinct trains of thought operating at one and the same time. He cannot prevent ideas of something awful about to happen, or as if he would do something awful. Imagine that they are being abused and energetically defend themselves against attacks and insults.

Mancinella: Delusion he will be taken by the devil. Delusion possessed.

Medorrhinum: Inclination to mutilate his body.

Mercurius: Inexpressive pain of soul and body, anxious restlessness, as if some evil impended, disgusted with himself. Has not the courage to live, constant suspicion, considering everybody his enemy.

Mandragora: Delusion he is possessed.

Moschus: Delusion she is dead.

Naja: As if under superhuman control. Antagonism with herself

Nitric acid: Delusion mind and body are separated; soul separated from his body. Hatred of those who have offended him.

Opium (narcotic polychrest): Delusion he is possessed; as if under superhuman control; of being possessed by two persons, of another self besides the real self—the opium man who does things which the real self considers wrong, and he is not always sure which will conquer the other. Antagonism with herself. Delusion he is dead. Sees animals coming toward him; people want to hurt him, execute him.

Paronichia illecebrum: Feeling that there are two different people inside him who contradict each other and argue about their illness. Doubling of personality.

Petroleum: Delusion body is divided. The whole day he is only half conscious, as if only half alive.

Phosphorus: Delusion as if seized; fancied he was in several pieces and could not get the fragments properly adjusted. Aversion to herself. Delusion he is dead.

Platina: Delusion she is possessed; as if under superhuman control. Aversion to herself. Delusions, pursued by ghosts.

Raphanus: Delusion he is dead. Sadness, aversion to children, especially girls. Nymphomania. Dangerous fancies assail her, but she restrains herself from putting them into execution.

Sabadilla: Delusions body and thoughts are separated. Delusion he is outside his body; mind and body are separated; soul separated from body.

Stramonium: Delusion body is divided; feet/hands are separated from the body. Delusion he is alive on one side and buried on the other. Strange absurd ideas—that he was killed, roasted, and being eaten. Delusion he is dead, pursued by ghosts. Inclination to mutilate his body. Constant vision of an executioner standing before him in spite of which he was lively, talkative, laughed and joked about his hallucination, yet it seemed to him a reality. Heard continually, on right side of occiput, a loud voice, scolding, vituperating and accusing him of ungodliness.

Thea: Sensations as if impelled by some uncontrollable power to commit suicide; jump out windows; kill her child. Nocturnal fright; sinister thoughts; invincible propensity to analyze his life, to look at it on the dark side, and to resolve it into its most hopeless realities.

Tarentula (spider polychrest): Self-torture; torments himself. Visions of monsters or animals that frighten him. Fear and shaking; the patient cannot find a suitable place where to hide himself; thinks he is going to be assaulted. Sudden foxlike destructive efforts, requiring utmost vigilance to prevent damage. Suddenly sprang away from her attendants and swept ornaments from mantelpiece; said she was sorry, but could not help it.

Thuja: Fixed idea—as if soul and body were separated—talks about being under the influence of a superior power. As if under superhuman control. Wants to be put in an insane asylum and treated harshly because she believes she has done wrong. Delusions, head belongs to another, body and thoughts are separated. Delusions cut in two, could not tell of which part had possession on waking; mind and body are separated. Contemptuous of self.

Remedies Made from Trees

TREES: abies-c. abies-n. abrom-a. acer-circ. acer-p. adans-d. aegle-f. aegle-m. aesc. aesc-c. aesc-g. agn. ail. aln, aln-g. alst. alst-s. amgd-p. amyg. anac. anac-oc. anders. ang. ango. anis. arb. arb-m. arb-u. asim. aza. bals.-p. bold. brach. bux. caj. camph. carp. cary. cas-s. casc. castn-v. cerc. cedr. cedrus-d. cedrus-l. celt. chin. chin-b. chion. choc. cinnm. coff. com. cop. corn-f. crat. crot-t. cupre-au. cupre-l. cyt-l. dat-a. dicha. dub. eryt-g. eucal. eucal-r. eucal-t. eug. euon. euon-a. eys. fic-c. fic-r. fic-v. frax. frax-e. frax-o. gamb. gink-b. gran. guaj. guar. guat. gymne. gymno. haem. ham. hura. hura-c. ign. ilx-a. ilx-c. ilx-v. jab. jac-c. jac-g. jatr-c. jatr-g. joan. jug-c. jug-r. juni-c. juni-o. juni-p. juni-v. just. just-r. kalm. kara. karw-h. kaur. kola. kurch. laur. magn-gl. magn-gr. manc. mangi. mate. melal. melal-alt-ol. musa. myric. myris. myrrha myrt-c. myrt-ch. myrt-p. neg. nux-a. nux-m nux-v. nyct. ol-sant. ol-su. olnd. oxyd. pana. paull. pers. pin-c. pin-l. pin-mo. pin-pa. pin-pi. pin-s. pisc. platan. platan-oc. platan- or. pop. pop-c. pop-n. prun. prun-am. prun-ar. prun-av. prun- cf. prun-cs. prun-d. prun-m. prun-p. prun-pe. prun-v. pseuts-m. ptel. pyrus. pyrus-c. quas. queb. quer. quill. rham-cal. rham-cath. rham-f. rham-pr. rhus-a. rhus-c. rhus-d. rhus-g. rhus-l. rhus-g. rhus-l. rhus-r. rhus-s. rhus-t. rhus-v. rhus-ver. ric. rob. sal-al. sal-am sal-fr. sal-l. sal-ma. sal-mo. sal-n. sal-p. samb. samb-c. samb-r. sap-o. sap-s. saroth. sass. seq-g. seq-s. soph. sorb-a. syr. syzyg. tama. tang. tax. tax-br. tere-ch. term-a. term-c. thea. thuj. thuj-g. thuj-l. til. til-al. til-ar. til-p. til-t. tong. ulm-c. ulm-m. ulm-pra. upa. upa-a. urt-g. vib. vib-l. vib-od. vib-p. vib-t. xan. yohim. yohim-m.

LARGE TREES: abies-c. abies-n. acer-p. adans-d. aesc. ail. aln-g. alst-s. anders. ango. arb-m. bals-p. camph. carp. cary. castn-v. cedrus-d. cedrus-l. celt. chin. china –b. cupre-au. cupre-l. eryt-g. eucal. eucal-r. eucal-t. frax. frax-e. frax-o. gink-b. gymno. hura. hura-c. jug-c. jug-r. juni-v. magn-gl. magn-gr. mangi. neg. nux-m. ol-su. oxyd. pers. pin-c. pin-l. pin-pa. pin-pi. pin-s. platan. platan-oc. platan-or. pop. pop-c. pop-n. prun-av. prun-v. pseuts-m. queb. quer. quill. rob. sal-al. sal-fr. sass. seq-g. seq-s. soph. sorb-a. syzyg. tama. tax. tere-ch. term-a. term-c. thuj. thuj-g. thuj-l. til. til-al. til-ar. til-p. til-t. tong. ulm-c. ulm-m. ulm-pra.

TREE-LIKE VINES: guar. gymne. paull. rhus-d. rhus-r. upa. upa-a.

CONIFERS: abies-c. abies-n. cedrus-d. cedrus-l. cop. cupre-au. cupre-l. juni-c. juni-o. juni-p. juni-v. ol-su. pin-c. pin-l. pin-mo. pin-pa. pin-pi. pin-s. pseuts-m. seq-g. seq-s. tax. tax-br. thuj. thuj-g. thuj-l.

ANCIENT TREES: adans-d. camph. cedrus-d. cedrus-l. cop. fic-r. gink-b. jug-r. kaur. magn-gr. ol-su. quer. seq-g. seq-s. til. til-al. til-ar. til-p. til-t.

Endnotes

CHAPTER ONE
Archetypal Dimensions of Healing

[1] David Bohm, *Wholeness and the Implicate Order* (London: Routledge Press, 1995), 1-2.

[2] Laurie Garret, *The Coming Plague: Newly Emerging Diseases in a World Out of Balance* (New York: Penguin Books, 1994), 620.

[3] Harris L. Coulter, *Divided Legacy: A History of the Schism in Medical Thought*, vol. 2 (Berkeley; California: North Atlantic Books, 1988), 703-704.

[4] C. G. Jung, *Psychology and Alchemy*, vol. 12 of *Collected Works of Carl Jung* (Princeton: Princeton University Press, 1993), 15.

[5] Ibid., 293.

[6] C. G. Jung, Mysterium Coniunctionis, vol. 14 of Collected Works of Carl Jung (Princeton: Princeton University Press, 1993), 228.

[7] Edward C. Whitmont, M.D., *The Alchemy of Healing: Psyche and Soma* (Berkeley, California: North Atlantic Books, 1993), 190-191.

[8] Adolf Guggenbühl-Craig, *Power in the Helping Professions* (Dallas: Spring Publications, 1992), 90.

[9] C. G. Jung, *Psychology and Alchemy*, vol. 12 of *Collected Works of Carl Jung* (Princeton: Princeton University Press, 1993), 228.

CHAPTER TWO
Homeopathy

[1] Harris L. Coulter, Divided Legacy: The Conflict Between Homoeopathy and the AMA (Berkeley, California: North Atlantic Books, 1975), 300-302.

[2] Dana Ullman, The Consumer's Guide to Homeopathy (New York: G. P. Putnam's Sons, 1995), 65.

[3] Dana Ullman, Homeopathic Family Medicine (an e-book) (Berkeley, California: www.homeopathic.com, first published: 2002, regularly updated).

[4] Paolo Bellavite, M.D., and Andrea Signorini, M.D., *The Emerging Science of Homeopathy: Complexity, Biodynamics, and Nanopharmacology* (Berkeley, California: North Atlantic Books, 2002), 77.

[5] George Vithoulkas, *The Science of Homeopathy* (New York: Grove, 1979).

[6] Taken from Stephen Hawking's Web site (www.hawking.org.uk/disable/dindex.html).

CHAPTER THREE

Psyche and Soma

[1] Alan B. Wallace, *Choosing Reality: A Buddhist View of Physics and the Mind* (Ithaca, New York: Snow Lion Publications, 1996), 40.

[2] Larry Dossey, M.D., *Reinventing Medicine: Beyond Mind-Body to a New Era of Healing* (San Francisco: HarperSanFrancisco, 1999), 191.

[3] V. Walter Odajnyk, *Gathering the Light, A Psychology of Meditation* (Boston: Shambhala, 1993), 42–46.

[4] *C. G. Jung,* The Practice of Psychotherapy, *vol. 16 of* Collected Works of Carl Jung *(Princeton: Princeton University Press, 1985), 330–337.*

[5] Samuel Hahnemann, *Organon of the Medical Art*, ed. Wenda B. O'Reilly (Redmond, Washington: Birdcage Books, 1996), 65.

[6] Edward C. Whitmont, *Psyche and Substance: Essays on Homeopathy in the Light of Jungian Psychology* (Berkeley, California: North Atlantic Books, 1980), 11.

CHAPTER FOUR

Archetypes and the Collective Unconscious

[1] Carl G. Jung, *Man and His Symbols* (New York: Doubleday, first published in 1964), 81–82.

[2] C. G. Jung, *The Structure and Dynamics of the Psyche*, vol. 8 of *Collected Works* (Princeton: Princeton University Press, 1981), 140.

[3] Marie-Louise von Franz, *Psyche and Matter* (Boston: Shambala Publications, 1992), 9.

[4] Ovid's *Metamorphosis*, Book VI, Pallas et Arachne, lines 1–213. Retold from *Bulfinch's Mythology* at www.bulfinch.org/fables/bull14.html.

[5] Massimo Mangialavori, M.D., and David Warkentin, P.A., *Spider Remedies*, Thema, Multimedia DVD. (Thema, Multimedia DVD).

CHAPTER FIVE

The Shadow

[1] C. G. Jung, *Aion*, vol. part 2 of *Collected Works of Carl Jung* (Princeton: Princeton University Press, 1978), 266.

[2] Ibid., 9.

[3] James Tyler Kent, A.M., M.D., *Lectures on Homeopathic Philosophy* (Berkeley, California: North Atlantic Books, 1979), 136.

[4] C. G. Jung, *Aion*, vol. 9 part 2 of *Collected Works of Carl Jung* (Princeton: Princeton University Press, 1978), 8.

CHAPTER SIX

Anima/Animus

[1] C. G. Jung, *The Archetypes and the Collective Unconscious*, vol. 9 of *collected Works of Carl Jung* Princeton: Princeton University Press, 1990), 29.

[2] Paracelsus, *The Hermetic and Alchemical Writings of Paracelsus*, ed. and trans. A. E. Waite (New Hyde Park: University Books, 1967), 1-153.

CHAPTER SEVEN

Wholeness

[1] C. G. Jung, *Man and His Symbols* (New York: Doubleday, first published in 1964), 166.

[2] C. G. Jung, *Psychology and Alchemy*, vol. 12 of *Collected Works of Carl Jung* (Princeton: Princeton University Press, 1993), 41.

[3] Jose and Miriam Arguelles, Mandala *(Boulder, Colorado: Shambala Publications, 1972), 91.*

[4] Edward F. Edinger, *Ego and Archetype* (Boston: Shambala Publications, 1992), 6.

[5] This original poem by Linda and her story are used with her permission, but her last name is withheld to protect her anonymity.

CHAPTER EIGHT

Dreams and the Mind-Body Relationship

[1] Samuel Hahnemann, *Organon of the Medical Art*, ed. Wenda Brewster O'Reilly (Redmond, Washington: Birdcage Books, 1996), 259.

[2] C. G. Jung, *Civilization in Transition*, vol. 10 of *Collected Works of Carl Jung* (Princeton: Princeton University Press, 1978), 144.

[3] Mircea Eliade, *Shamanism: Archaic Techniques of Ecstasy* (Princeton: Princeton University Press, 1974), 39.

[4] C. G. Jung, *The Archetypes and the Collective Unconscious*, vol. 9 of *Collected Works of Carl Jung* (Princeton: Princeton University Press, 1990), 169.

[5] C. G. Jung, *The Practice of Psychotherapy*, vol. 16 of *Collected Works of Carl Jung* (Princeton: Princeton University Press, 1985), 158-160.

[6] Ibid., 160.

CHAPTER NINE

Case Taking

[1] Suggested reading on Jungian Typology:

> C. G. Jung, *Psychological Types*, vol. 6 of *Collected Works of Carl Jung* (Princeton: Princeton University Press, 1974).

> Marie Louise von Franz and James Hillman, *Lectures on Jung's Typology* (Woodstock: Spring Publications, 1998).

Daryl Sharp, *Personality Types: Jung's Model of Typology* (Toronto: Inner City Books, 1987).

Calvin S. Hall and Gardner Lindsey, *Theories of Personality* (New York: John Wiley & Sons, Inc., 1970).

[2] C. G. Jung, *The Practice of Psychotherapy*, vol. 16 of *Collected Works of Carl Jung* (Princeton: Princeton University Press, 1985), 218.

[3] *The I Ching or Book of Changes*, trans. Richard Wilhelm, Bollingen Foundation (Princeton: Princeton University Press, 1967), 194.

[4] Edward C. Whitmont, M.D., *The Alchemy of Healing: Psyche and Soma* (Berkeley, California: North Atlantic Books, 1993), 189.

[5] Adolf Guggenbühl-Craig, *Power in the Helping Professions* (Dallas: Spring Publications, 1992), 38–39.

Chapter Ten
Communicating with the Psyche

[1] Shunryu Suzuki, *Zen Mind, Beginner's Mind* (New York: Weatherhill, Inc., 1994), 21.

[2] John Chevalier and Alain Gheerbrant, *The Penguin Dictionary of Symbols* (New York: Penguin Books USA, 1994).

[3] C. G. Jung, *The Symbolic Life*, vol. 18 of *Collected Works of Carl Jung* (Princeton: Princeton University Press, 1989), 207.

[4] Ibid., p. 210.

[5] Samuel Hahnemann, *Materia Medica Pura*, vol. 1 (New Delhi: B. Jain Publishers, reprinted 1986), 458.

[6] C. G. Jung, *The Symbolic Life*, vol. 18 of *Collected Works of Carl Jung* (Princeton: Princeton University Press, 1989), 214.

[7] Ibid., 215.

Part IV
Symbolic Materia Medica

[1] From *Secret Symbols of the Rosecrucians*. This eighteenth-century compendium drew on seventeenth-century alchemical sources such as Adrian von Mynsich, with mystical pieces from Valentin Weigel, and Abraham von Franckenberg's works on Jacob Boehme.

Chapter Eleven
Trees

[1] C. G. Jung, Collected Alchemical Studies, vol. 13 of *Collected Works of Carl Jung* (Princeton: Princeton University Press, 1983), 272.

[2] From van Gogh's letters, translated by R. G. Harrison (www.vangoghgallery.com letters/main.htm).

³ I have retold this story. The original can be found on the Maori website http://www.maori.org.nz/tikanga/purakau/creation.htm.

⁴ Source: School of Homeopathy website http://www.hominf.org.uk/kaur/kaurintr.htm#Remedy.

⁵ Mircea Eliade, *Shamanism: Archaic Techniques of Ecstasy* (Princeton: Princeton University Press, 1964), 272.

⁶ Timothy F. Allen, *Encyclopedia of Pure Materia Medica,* vol. 2 (New Delhi: B. Jain Publishers), 424-425.

⁷ Samuel Hahnemann, *Materia Medica Pura,* vol. 1 (New Delhi: B. Jain Publishers, reprinted), 304.

⁸ I've retold this story from *Myth and Mankind Series / Lost Realms of Gold: South American Myth* (Amsterdam: Time-Life Books, 1998), 31.

⁹ Jeremy Scherr, *The Homeopathic Proving of Chocolate* (Northampton: Dynamis School for Advanced Homeopathic Studies, n.d.), 67.

¹⁰ C. G. Jung, *Symbols of Transformation,* vol. 5 in *Collected Works of Carl Jung* (Princeton: Princeton University Press, 1990), 351.

¹¹ Retold from *Bulfinch's Mythology,* Chapter VI, "Baucis and Philemon," http://www.webcom.com/shownet/bulfinch/fables/bull6.html.

¹² Robert Bannan, "A Proving of Tilia Cordata," *Homeopathic Links* 9 (Summer 1996): 104.

CHAPTER TWELVE

Vines

¹ Eihei Dogen, *Moon in a Dewdrop, Writings of Zen Master Dogen,* ed. Kazuaki Tanahashi (New York, North Point Press, 1985), 168-174.

² Ibid., 169.

³ Clair Dunne, *Carl Jung: Wounded Healer of the Soul* (New York: Parabola Books, 2000), 210.

CHAPTER THIRTEEN

Milk Symbolism

¹ The story of Romulus and Remus is about children who, without bonding to a natural parent, are raised by an animal. **The complete version of my very brief retelling of Plutarch's story of Romulus can be found on the Internet Classics Archive at http://classics.mit.edu/Plutarch/romulus.html.

² Michael Maier's alchemical emblem book Atalanta Fugiens was first published in Latin in 1617. It incorporated fifty emblems, each with a motto, an epigram, and a discourse; the book also included fifty pieces of music the 'fugues' or canons. They can be seen and heard on this Web site (www.levity.com/alchemy/home.html).

³ James Tyler Kent, *Lectures on Homeopathic Materia Medica* (New Delhi: Homeopathic Publications, Reprinted), 612.

[4] C. G. Jung, *Symbols of Transformation,* vol. 5 of Collected Works of Carl Jung (Princeton: Princeton University Press, 1990), 297.

[5] Karl-Josef Mueller and Gerhard Ruster, Lac Felinum: A Synthetic Remedy Picture (Zwibrucken: Private Publication, 1995).

[6] Marie-Louise von Franz, *The Cat: A Tale of Feminine Redemption* (Toronto: Inner City Books, 1999).

[7] Ibid., 60.

[8] Alize Timmerman, "The Symbol in a Remedy as a Key Factor," *Homeopathic Links* 9 (1996): 148–150.

[9] Anne Wirtz, "A Caring Capricious Creature, Lac Felinum," Homeopathic Links 9 (1996): 145–148.

[10] *New Larousse Encyclopedia of Mythology,* s.v. "Hathor." (London, The Hamlyn Publishing Group Limited, 1959)

[11] Jean Chevalier and Alain Gheerbrant, *The Penguin Dictionary of Symbols* (New York: Penguin Books, 1996), 237.

CHAPTER FOURTEEN
The Seven Metals of the Alchemists

[1] Samuel Hahnemann, *Materia Medica Pura,* vol. 1 (New Delhi: B. Jain Publishers, reprinted), 180.

[2] James Tyler Kent, *Lectures on Homeopathic Materia Medica* (New Delhi: Homeopathic Publications), 787.

[3] Timothy F. Allen, M.D., *The Encyclopedia of Pure Materia Medica,* vol. 9 (New Delhi: B. Jain Publishers), 129.

[4] Samuel Hahnemann, *Materia Medica Pura,* vol. 1 (New Delhi: B. Jain Publishers), 180.

CHAPTER FIFTEEN
The Internal Saboteur

[1] Donald Kalsched, *The Inner World of Trauma: Archetypal Defenses of the Personal Spirit* (New York: Routledge Press, 1996). 4.

[2] Ibid., 5.

[3] Constantine Hering, M.D., *The Guiding Symptoms of our Materia Medica,* vol. 10 (New Delhi: B. Jain Publishers), 159–166.

[4] Donald Kalsched, *The Inner World of Trauma: Archetypal Defenses of the Personal Spirit* (New York: Routledge Press, 1996).

[5] C. G. Jung, *Mysterium Coniunctionis,* vol. 14 of Collected Works of Carl Jung (Princeton: Princeton University Press, 1989), 155.

[6] John Henry Clarke, M.D., *A Dictionary of Practical Materia Medica,* vol. 1 (New Delhi: Jain Publishing Co. Reprinted), 69.

[7] Frans Vermeulen, *Synoptic Materia Medica II* (Haarlem: Merlijn Publishers, 1996), 13.

[8] John Henry Clarke, M.D., *A Dictionary of Practical Materia Medica*, vol. 1 (New Delhi: Jain Publishing), 5.

[9] Bruno Marinez, M.D., "Folliculinum: Efficacy in Premenstrual Syndrome," British Homoeopathic Journal, vol. 79, (April 1990): 104-105.

[10] Dorothy Cooper, "Folliculinum," British Homoeopathic Journal, vol. 79 (April 1990): 100.

[11] Timothy F. Allen, M.D., *The Encyclopedia of Pure Materia Medica*, vol. 5 (New Delhi: B. Jain Publishers), 573.

[12] Ibid., 571.

Glossary of Jungian and Alchemical Terms

active imagination

The use of a dream or some other fantasy image or mood in order to explore different parts of the personality. The mind is concentrated on the mind object or mood, which activates and animates it. These alterations are then carefully noted, because they reflect the psychic processes in the unconscious. Active imagination is a powerful tool for uniting the conscious and unconscious.

anima

The inner feminine side of a man. Jung called the anima, a man's soul, as, ultimately, she helps the man connect with the archetypal realms of the psyche. The anima can be a creative muse, but her negative aspect can lead him into the realms of fantasy, especially when it comes to relationships with women.

animus

The inner masculine side of a woman. The negative animus may act as an inner critic and stand in the way of a woman's accomplishments. On the other hand, she may be driven by such an animus to the degree that she loses her femininity. The positive animus serves as a spiritual guide and helps a woman be successful in life.

archetype

The unconscious and innate predispositions that make up the collective unconscious. The archetype itself is invisible but stimulates the formation of imagery that results in archetypal symbols. Although the origin of the archetypes cannot be understood except by conjecture, they appear to be related to basic human needs and instincts. Jung felt that they were inherent within the brain structure.

collective unconscious

A part of the psyche containing elements inherited from generations of human consciousness. A distinction must be made with the personal unconscious that pertains to the individual. However, as the contents of the personal unconscious are made conscious, the images and symbols of the collective unconscious are revealed.

complex

The source of negative emotions, complexes are the essential components of the psyche and the source of greater effort and achievement.

coniunctio

A term borrowed by Jung from alchemy. It originally referred to the chemical combination of elements, but is used in psychology to refer to the union of opposites within the psyche and subsequent birth of new possibilities.

countertransference

A term used to describe the projection of the therapist's unconscious emotional responses onto the patient. Jung called this mutual unconsciousness one of the chief occupational hazards of psychotherapy. Countertransference applies, however, not only to the psychotherapeutic relationship but may occur in any doctor-patient relationship.

ego

The central complex of consciousness. Jung felt that the ego develops partly by inherited predispositions and is partly acquired. An understanding of the contents of the ego is often confused with self-understanding. However, the ego can only know its own contents and not the unconscious.

Eros

In mythology, Eros is the personification of love. Eros also represents the instinctual, animal nature. It is the capacity to relate to others. Jung felt that unconscious Eros always expresses itself as a will to power.

extraversion

Orientation toward the outer world. The psychic energy of the extravert naturally moves outward onto people and his or her environment. Data from this outside world is the primary source for the individual's decisions and behaviors.

feeling

The psychological function that evaluates or judges the worth of things or people. It is not, however, to be confused with emotion.

function

A form of psychic activity that remains the same under all conditions. Jung's model of typology includes thinking and feeling, which are considered to be rational functions and sensation and intuition, considered to be irrational functions.

individuation

The process of psychological differentiation that develops the individual personality. The goal of individuation is to leave behind false wrappings of the persona on one hand, and to free oneself from the grip of primordial images on the other.

inferior function

The least developed, therefore the most primitive, function in an individual. In some, the inferior function may fall into the unconscious and give rise to infantile desires or other symptoms of neurosis.

inflation

An exaggerated and overblown state of mind. It is an unconscious state that renders us incapable of learning from the past, understanding events in the present, and drawing right conclusions about the future. Inflation is a sign for the need to assimilate unconscious complexes.

introversion

A psychological orientation in which the movement of energy is toward the inner state. Introverts are motivated primarily by their inner world and receive energy from being alone.

intuition

The psychological function that gives insight based on information from the inner state or from subliminal perceptions of outer awareness. In any case, intuitive knowledge possesses an intrinsic certainty and conviction. Jung considered it to be an irrational function.

Logos

Logic and structure. Logos is the ability for discrimination, judgment, and insight and is associated in Jungian psychology with spirit.

mandala

The magic circle used in many cultures. It was seen by Jung as a symbol of the Self, wholeness, and psychological balance. He came to this idea after seeing Eastern mandalas that were used for meditation. The alchemical vessel is a counterpart to the mandala.

Mercurius

Considered by the alchemists to be the spirit imprisoned in matter, to be freed through the alchemical process. Also known as Hermes, he stands for the prima material, or beginning of the work, and the goal, or philosopher's stone.

myth
A tale, fable, or motif that unconsciously symbolizes the activities of the collective unconscious. Myths aren't created, they arise from the unconscious and serve as mediators between the unconscious and conscious states.

numinous
Referring the feeling of mystery, terror, and fascination associated with an encounter with a presence greater than ordinary reality. Jung refers to contact with archetypal energies as numinous.

persona
Originally meaning a mask that is worn by an actor, the persona is a protective personality that is worn in order to adapt and get along in society. It is an asset in interacting with other people, and society depends upon interactions through the persona. A problem only occurs when the individual identifies with the persona and is unable to rid himself or herself of this artificial personality at will.

personal unconscious
That aspect of the unconscious that contains personal memories, repressed ideas and subliminal perceptions. It is individual and distinct from the collective unconscious.

philosopher's stone
Also known as the lapis philosophorum or ultima materia, it was supposed to grant immortality, heal all disease, and transform base metals into gold. To Jung, it represented the Self and the goal of individuation.

prima materia
An alchemical term meaning "original matter," from which the alchemists attempted to create the philosopher's stone. The term is used in Jungian psychology to represent the whole of undifferentiated material that must be sorted through in analysis.

primary function
Also known as the superior function, it is the individual's most developed function. As a general rule, a person identifies strongly with their primary function and it continues to dominate his or her other functions throughout his or her life.

Self
The archetype of wholeness. The Self is a regulating aspect of the psyche that transcends the ego. The realization of the Self is always at the expense of the ego as it dwarfs it in scope and intensity.

sensation function
The psychological function that perceives through the senses without judgment as to their worth or meaning. Jung considered sensation to be an irrational function.

shadow
Aspects of the individual that have been repressed or never recognized. The shadow may contain much that is useful but for some reason has not been accepted by the individual or by society. Becoming conscious of the shadow means recognizing the dark and unacknowledged aspect of the personality.

symbol
Imagery and ideas that are an expression for something unknown and point toward greater reality. Jung differentiated between a symbol and a sign. A sign, he said, is a symbol whose meaning is specifically defined.

synchronicity
Defined by Jung as an "acausal connecting principle," it represents the mysterious connection between the personal psyche and the material world. It is where the outside world coincides with a psychological state in a meaningful way.

thinking function
A mode of psychological functioning based on the mental process of interpreting what is perceived. Jung considered it to be a rational function.

transference
A phenomenon in which unconscious contents are projected upon persons and situations. Although it may occur in almost any situation, it is typically used to refer to the projection of a patients unconscious feelings onto the therapist. Projections can be either positive or negative and most relationships are made up in large part by projection.

transcendent function
A function that arises from the tension between the unconscious and the conscious mind and supports their union. Development of the transcendent function depends upon becoming aware of unconscious material, which is accomplished through dream analysis and active imagination.

vas hermeticum
The alchemical retort in which the alchemist cooked the prima materia into the lapis. It was often made of glass, and it was important for it to be round like the cosmos.

Bibliography

Homeopathy

Allen, Henry C. *The Materia Medica with the Nosodes and Provings of X-Ray.* Reprint, New Delhi: B. Jain Publishers.

Allen, Timothy F., M.D. *The Encyclopedia of Pure Materia Medica.* Reprint, New Delhi: B. Jain Publishers.

Bannan, Robert. "A Proving of Tilia Cordata." Homeopathic Links 9 (Summer 1996): 104.

Bellavite, Paolo, M.D., and Andrea Signorini, M.D. *The Emerging Science of Homeopathy: Complexity, Biodynamics, and Nanopharmacology.* Berkeley, California: North Atlantic Books, 2002.

Clarke, John Henry, M.D. *A Dictionary of Practical Materia Medica,* vol. 1. Reprint, New Delhi: Jain Publishing Co, 1982.

Cooper, Dorothy. "Folliculinum." British Homoeopathic Journal, vol. 79 (April 1990): 100.

Coulter, Harris L. *Divided Legacy: A History of the Schism in Medical Thought,* vol. 2. Berkeley, California: North Atlantic Books, 1988.

Hahnemann, Samuel. *Materia Medica Pura.* Reprint, New Delhi: B. Jain Publishers, 1986.

———, *Organon of the Medical Art.* Ed. Wenda B. O'Reilly. Redmond, Washington: Birdcage Books, 1996.

Hering, Constantine, M.D. *The Guiding Symptoms of Our Materia Medica.* Reprint, New Delhi: B. Jain Publishers.

Kent, James Tyler. *Lectures on Homeopathic Materia Medica.* Reprint, New Delhi: Homeopathic Publications.

———. *Lectures on Homeopathic Philosophy.* 1900. Reprint with forward by Dana Ullman, Berkeley, California: North Atlantic Books, 1979.

Mangialavori, Massimo, M.D., and David Warkentin, PA. Spider Remedies. Thema, Multimedia DVD.

Marinez Bruno, M.D. "Folliculinum: Efficacy in Premenstrual Syndrome." British Homoeopathic Journal, vol. 79 (April 1990): 104-105.

Mueller, Karl-Josef and Gerhard Ruster. Lac Felinum: A Synthetic Remedy Picture. Zwibrucken: Private Publication, 1995.

Scholten, Jan, M.D. *Homeopathy and the Elements.* Netherlands: Stiching Alonnissos, 1996.

Sherr, Jeremy. *The Homeopathic Proving of Chocolate.* Northampton: Dynamis School for Advanced Homeopathic Studies, n.d.

Timmerman, Alize. "The Symbol in a Remedy as a Key Factor." Homeopathic Links 9 (1996): 148-150.

Ullman, Dana. *The Consumer's Guide to Homeopathy.* New York: G.P. Putnam's Sons, 1995.

——. *Homeopathic Family Medicine* (an e-book). Berkeley, California: www.homeopathic.com, First published: 2002, regularly updated.

Vermeulen, Frans. *Synoptic Materia Medica II.* Haarlem: Merlign Publishers, 1996.Vithoulkas, George. *The Science of Homeopathy.* New York: Grove, 1979.

Whitmont, Edward C., M.D. *The Alchemy of Healing: Psyche and Soma.* Berkeley, California: North Atlantic Books, 1993.

——. *Psyche and Substance: Essays on Homeopathy in the Light of Jungian Psychology.* Berkeley, California: North Atlantic Books, 1980.

Wirtz, Anne. "A Caring Capricious Creature, Lac Felinum." Homeopathic Links 9 (1996): 145-148.

Zanvandervoort, Roger. *The Complete Repertory.* version 4.5 CDRom, Institute for Research in Homeopathic Information and Symptomology.

Jungian Psychology

Boa, Fraser. *The Way of the Dream: Conversations on Jungian Dream Interpretation with Marie-Louise von Franz.* Boston: Shambhala Publications, 1992.

Dunne, Claire. *Carl Jung: Wounded Healer of the Soul.* New York: Parabola Books, 2000.

Edinger, Edward F. *Anatomy of the Psyche: Alchemical Symbolism in Psychotherapy.* La Salle, Illinois: Open Court, 1994.

——. *Ego and Archetype.* Shambhala Publications: Boston, 1992.

Guggenbühl-Craig, Adolf. *Power in the Helping Professions.* Dallas: Spring Publications, 1992. Jung, C. G. Collected Works, (Bollingen Series XX). Trans. R. F. C. Hull. 20 vols. Princeton: Princeton University Press, 1976-1993.

——. *Symbols of Transformation,* vol. 5 of Collected Works of Carl Jung. Princeton: Princeton University Press, 1990.

——. *Psychological Types,* vol. 6 of Collected Works of Carl Jung. Princeton: Princeton University Press, 1974.

——. *The Structure and Dynamics of the Psyche,* vol. 8 of Collected Works of Carl Jung. Princeton: Princeton University Press, 1981.

——. *The Archetypes and the Collective Unconscious,* vol. 9 of Collected Works of Carl Jung. Princeton: Princeton University Press, 1990.

——. *Aion,* vol. 9 part 2 of Collected Works of Carl Jung. Princeton: Princeton University Press, 1978.

——. *Civilization in Transition,* vol. 10 of Collected Works of Carl Jung. Princeton: Princeton University Press, 1978.

——. *Psychology and Alchemy,* vol. 12 of Collected Works of Carl Jung. Princeton: Princeton University Press, 1993.

——. *Alchemical Studies,* vol. 13 of Collected Works of Carl Jung. Princeton: Princeton University Press, 1983.

——. *Mysterium Coniunctionis,* vol. 14 of Collected Works of Carl Jung. Princeton: Princeton University Press, 1993

——. *The Practice of Psychotherapy,* vol. 16 of Collected Works of Carl Jung. Princeton: Princeton University Press, 1985.

——. *The Symbolic Life,* vol. 18 of Collected Works of Carl Jung. Princeton: Princeton University Press, 1989.

——. *Dream Analysis,* Notes of the Seminar Given in 1928-1930 by C. G. Jung, (Bollingen Series XCIX). Ed. Wm. McGuire. Princeton: Princeton University Press, 1984.

——. *Man and His Symbols.* New York: Doubleday, first published in 1964.

——. *Memories, Dreams and Reflections.* Ed. Aniela Jaffe. New York: Vintage Books, 1989.

Jung, Emma. *Anima and Animus.* Dallas: Spring Publications, Inc. 1985.

Kalsched, Donald. *The Inner World of Trauma: Archetypal Defenses of the Personal Psyche.* New York: Routledge, 1996.

Sharp, Daryl. *Personality Types: Jung's Model of Typology.* Toronto: Inner City Books, 1987.

——. *C. G. Jung Lexicon: A Primer of Terms & Concepts.* Toronto: Inner City Books, 1991.

von Franz, Marie-Louise. *Alchemical Active Imagination.* Boston: Shambhala Publications, 1997.

——. *Archetypal Dimensions of the Psyche.* Boston: Shambhala Publications, 1999.

——. *Alchemy: An Introduction to the Symbolism and the Psychology.* Toronto: Inner City Books, 1980.

——. *The Cat: A Tale of Feminine Redemption.* Toronto: Inner City Books, 1999.

——. *Projection and Re-collection in Jungian Psychology: Reflections of the Soul.* Chicago: Open Court, 1995.

——. *Psyche and Matter.* Boston: Shambhala Publications, 1992.

von Franz, Marie-Louise, and James Hillman. *Lectures on Jung's Typology.* Woodstock, New York: Spring Publications, Inc., 1998.

Mythology, Symbolism, and Spirituality

Arguelles, Jose and Miriam. *Mandala.* Boulder: Shambala Publications, 1972.

Chevalier, Jean and Alain Gheerbrant. *A Dictionary of Symbols.* Trans. John Buchanan-Brown. London: Penguin Books, 1996.

Dogen, Eihei. *Moon in a Dewdrop: Writings of Zen Master Dogen*. Ed. Kazuaki Tanahashi. New York: North Point Press, 1985.

Eliade, Mircea. *Images and Symbols: Studies in Religious Symbolism*. Princeton: Princeton University Press, 1991.

——. *Myths, Dreams, and Mysteries*. New York: Harper & Row, 1967.

——. *Shamanism: Archaic Techniques of Ecstasy* (Bollingen Series LXXVI). Trans. Willard R. Trask. Princeton: Princeton University Press, 1974.

Odajnyk, V. Walter. *Gathering the Light: A Psychology of Meditation*. Boston: Shambhala Publications, 1993.

Ovid's *Metamorphosis*, Book VI. Pallas et Arachne. www.bulfinch.org/fables/bull14.html

Roseman, Marina. *Healing Sounds from the Malaysian Rain Forest: Temiar Music and Medicine*. Berkeley, California: University of California Press, 1993.

Suzuki, Shunryu. *Zen Mind, Beginner's Mind*. New York: Weatherhill, Inc., 1994.

Time-Life Books, *Myth and Mankind Series/Lost Realms of Gold: South American Myth*. Amsterdam: Time-Life Books, 1998.

Underhill, Evelyn. *Mysticism: The Nature and Development of Spiritual Consciousness*. Oxford: Oneworld Publications, 2000.

Wallace, Alan B. *Choosing Reality: A Buddhist View of Physics and the Mind*. Ithaca, New York: Snow Lion Publications, 1996.

Wilhelm, Richard, trans. *The I Ching or Book of Changes*. Princeton: Princeton University Press, 1967.

Other

Bohm, David. *Wholeness and the Implicate Order*. London: Routledge Press, 1995.

Dossey, Larry, M.D. *Reinventing Medicine: Beyond Mind-Body to a New Era of Healing*. San Francisco: HarperSanFrancisco, 1999.

Garret, Laurie. *The Coming Plague: Newly Emerging Diseases in a World Out of Balance*. New York: Penguin Books, 1994.

Index

About the Author

Jane Cicchetti RSHom(NA), CCH, has been a consultant and teacher of homeopathy for twenty years. She is Director of the Five Elements School of Homeopathy in New Jersey, and teaches regularly on dreams and symbols in homeopathy to medical professionals in the U.S. and Holland. Her most recent course, Dreams, Symbols, and the Healing Process, integrates Jung's work on dream symbolism and alchemy into classical homeopathy.

Ms. Cicchetti has had a life-long interest in meditation and transpersonal psychology. She is a student of Zen meditation and has studied Jungian psychology under the mentorship of a Jungian analyst for the last ten years.

8/28 - Th
8/29 - Fri
9/2 - Tues
9/8 - Mon
9/9 - Tues
9/15 - Mon
9/16 - Tues

Fandango Dispute

bankofamerica billing inquires
@ PO Box 982234
El Paso, TX 79998

Fax = 302 457 8346